Foraging Medicinal Plants of New England

How to safely identify and prepare over 100 medicinal plants for herbal remedies

Silvi Pavlova

© Copyright 2022 - All rights reserved.

The content contained within this book may not be reproduced, duplicated or transmitted without direct written permission from the author or the publisher.

Under no circumstances will any blame or legal responsibility be held against the publisher, or author, for any damages, reparation, or monetary loss due to the information contained within this book, either directly or indirectly.

Legal Notice:

This book is copyright protected. It is only for personal use. You cannot amend, distribute, sell, use, quote, or paraphrase any part of the content within this book, without the consent of the author or publisher.

Disclaimer Notice:

Please note the information contained within this document is for educational and entertainment purposes only. All effort has been expended to present accurate, up-to-date, reliable, and complete information. No warranties of any kind are declared or implied. Readers acknowledge that the author is not engaged in the rendering of legal, financial, medical, or professional advice. The content within this book has been derived from various sources. Please consult a licensed professional before attempting any techniques outlined in this book.

By reading this document, the reader agrees that under no circumstances is the author responsible for any losses, direct or indirect, that are incurred as a result of the use of the information contained within this document, including, but not limited to, errors, omissions, or inaccuracies.

Contents

Introduction	1
1. Natural Health Through Healing Herbs—An Essential Primer	7
2. Chapter 2: Profiles of Medicinal Plants in New England	17
Woody - Trees	23
Woody - Bushes/Shrubs	43
Woody -Liana (Woody Vines)	58
Herbaceous - Graminoids (Grasses)	62
Herbaceous - Forb (Flowering)	65
Herbaceous - Fern	87
3. Creating Your Own Herbal Remedies Part One: Basic Processes and Techniques	88
4. Creating Your Own Herbal Remedies Part Two: Modes of Preparation	97
5. Creating Your Own Herbal Remedies Part Three: Recipes	108
Remedies for Allergies	110

Remedies for Respiratory Ailments	113
Remedies for Maintaining Wellness	116
Remedies for Digestive Problems	120
Remedies for Stress and Anxiety	125
Remedies for Beauty Care	129
Remedies for Inflammation	134
Remedies for Minor Wounds and Bruises	136
Remedies for Regulating Blood Pressure	140
Remedies for Treating Infections	142
Remedies for Bloating	146
Remedies for Insect Bites, Stings, and Rashes	149
Other Remedies	154
6. Foraging for Medicinal Herbs in New England	158
7. Cultivating Medicinal Plants at Home	165
Conclusion	175
References	177

Get The Ultimate Healthy Living Book Bundle

4 practical guides to help you use herbs as healing tools

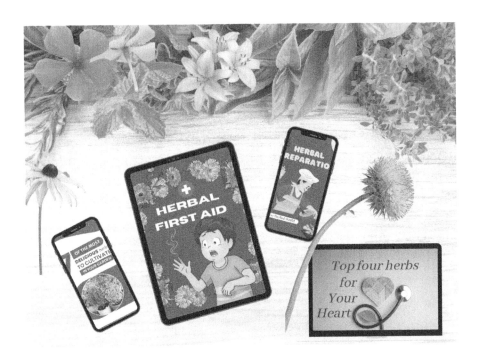

1. The Herbal First Aid – always be prepared for emergencies:
2. The Top Four Herbs for Your Heart guide
3. 7 Delicious Herbs to Cultivate in Your Garden
4. The Herbal Preparation Guide

Just scan the QR code or go to
https://goherbalworld.com/

BONUS: 1. Get your own Harvesting/Wildcrafting Calendar to print or use as your desktop wallpaper to always know what's fresh!

BONUS: 2. All illustrations from the book (copyright reserved)

And this is not all.

On the Go Herbal World web page, you can find much more!

We hub a search button where you can find all benefits, uses for, harvest times, and dangers (if there are any) of all herbs included in this book.

Introduction

The treatment process between pharmaceutical medication and plant-based medicine is not as different as it may seem. Melatonin (N-acetyl-5-methoxytryptamine), commonly known as a sleep aid, is also found in many plants such as Tanacetum parthenium, more commonly known as Feverfew. The benefits of pharmaceutical medication are undeniable. Its sophisticated formulas, exact dosage, and its ability to target complex health issues will always be necessary for treating ailments. Just the same, herbal treatments have their place as well. This being so, people are returning to these natural ingredients more and more for their healing abilities. Done right, common cold symptoms can be dealt with at home with locally sourced plants. These are cost-effective and natural treatment options. This book is focused on creating accessibility to these realistic and accurate home remedies.

The community formed from a shared interest in healing plants and remedies is diverse, both in personal background and in their motivation for discovering more about local plant properties. Religion and spirituality, physical and mental health, the increase in both pharmaceutical price and distrust, reconnection with their environment/environmental anxiety, or even simply fascination interest, begins the ever-expanding, extensive list of reasons for taking a more hands-on approach to healing.

Because of the growing interest in plant-based remedies, it has begun to shed its image as a lost art or mysterious hocus-pocus. No longer is it just a fringe alternative, it is a mainstream choice. Whatever your personal reason for exploring medicinal herbalism, everyone is welcome and encouraged to take their place here.

Besides herbal remedies, the ability to obtain a way of life that is more self-sufficient and less industrially reliant grows as well. *Urban Foraging and the Relational Ecologies*, a study focused on foraging in Seattle, discusses the relationship people have with foraging to connect with their cultures and create a "place" for people, even in cities (Poe et al., 2014). This reconnection with the wild alleviates anxieties by giving agency to people in a world of mounting industrialization, giving city dwellers the ability to create a more complex relationship with food and blurring the lines between the urban and the wild (Poe et al., 2014). Foraging takes us beyond socio-historical-political-economic factors, as it's something simple and deeply human. In addition to foraging for foods in both cities and country scapes, in this book, we will work on building tools to give you knowledge on identifying and harvesting plants; cultivating your own garden; and creating tried-and-true recipes. These skills will allow you to create a deeper relationship/understanding between you and your environment, in addition to the other personal reasons you might be practicing herbal medicine.

The world of foraging, remedies, gardening, and beyond may seem like individualistic hobbies, but there is a united effort for responsible growing and harvesting. Because of isolation, getting into alternative medicine can be a hurdle. Without accessible resources, it is easy to become overwhelmed or discouraged by inaccurate, overwhelming, outdated, non-specific, or irrelevant reiterations of information. Plenty of my time spent in this field has been spent weeding out false claims from the fact-based ones—giving respect and believability back to the alternative community. Sometimes this can be extremely tiresome, as we are unable to determine who has the authority to talk on these subjects. Taking a realistic and responsible approach to this journey is the best and only way to reap the benefits of plant-based remedies and herbal-based living. Herbalism has long been practiced using knowledge passed down from generation to generation and has always been a community effort to share effective treatments.

My own interest in herbalism was bound to happen after living in the countryside, being surrounded by a plethora of plants. When I was a child, I had a condition where clumps of my hair would fall out regularly. The doctors my mom brought me to were never able to find the real cause. But thankfully my family is a big believer in the power of herbal remedies. I would often accompany my grandfather to go foraging for herbs in the forests near our home. My mom made sure that healing herbs were part of my regular diet. She made a concoction from nettle that she would often apply to my scalp. Well, here I am today and my hair has never been stronger, shinier, or more beautiful.

My parents' accumulation of plant knowledge often filled in the gaps for the many questions I had. Still, it fascinated me that plants like poison ivy could cover me in a rash for weeks, but only a few strides up the path could be a delicious raspberry bush. This leads to the obvious next question—what do all the plants in between do? Are we missing out on the plant that grows in between the cracks in the pavement? Once I started putting words and meanings to the endless dictionary of plants, the world slowly became more magical. "Flower" wasn't enough when passing a garden. Careful observation of the difference between daisies and chamomile, for example, and further understanding that their properties are calming, anti-inflammatory and digestive, created an appreciation for the wild that comes with identification.

I started collecting and drying plants I had identified as medicinal, but eventually came to have a very large inventory and did not know what to do with it. I was jarring and preserving food from my grandma's garden at this point, and knew that there was more that I could do with the herbs than simply use dried leaves for tea. The first thing I made was a simple salve from pine resin, beeswax, and olive oil (anti-bacterial, anti-fungal properties for cuts and bruises.) Since then, I have worked to continually extend my knowledge about plant-based therapies, reaping the benefits of improved health, which I have found is better obtained through the addition of plant-based remedies.

The most effective tip for using these natural remedies is understanding that they are not magic, nor are they miracles. Someone who has regular seasonal allergies might be able to create a slow immunity by eating local honey to introduce your body to these foreign bodies. Seasonal allergies tend to be caused by whatever pollen is in the air. The idea is that bees in your local area use this same pollen to make honey. Allergies are the body's reaction to something it doesn't know, so slowly getting used to pollen from plants typically native to your area can stop the body from reacting as severely.

Alongside this treatment, these people might use anti-inflammatory teas to relieve symptoms. This might be instead of, in addition to or as the first step before using over-the-counter antihistamines. If you are someone who needs an EpiPen due to extreme allergic reactions, these treatments are not going to be effective. It is important to know when you need a Band-aid and when you need stitches. Herbal remedies are meant to be used for treating daily symptoms you might experience, such as dry skin, digestive issues, sleeping issues, and so on. Living a healthy life is a combination of everything you do and adding herbal remedies can be a great tool to become a well-rounded person. It is an addition to your life.

Getting into Herbalism

By following carefully curated, accurate, and understandable information, you will be able to apply this knowledge to deal with health issues. You will be able to use alternative herbal-based medicine to move away from dependency on commercial solutions. For optimal results, my recommendation is to read this book in a linear fashion first. It is a field guide, meaning that you can flip to identification or recipes as you need them, but take the time to get familiar with all the information, and where it is, before jumping into action. Each of these different topics is intertwined. The mystery around plant-based medicine is partly erased by understanding what the process looks like before you start it. Accurate healing can only be achieved when you understand the intentions and reasons behind each step. Understanding also means safe foraging, dosing, and mixing of herbs .

Chapter 7 looks at cultivating your own garden. Getting a grasp on the way these things intersect with your practice will set you up for success from the start.

chapter, we will go deeper into what it means to use natural healing methods. This includes history and the resurgence of herbal medicine, and what that means for practitioners in the world of conventional healing. The chapter is unabashed about critical questions such as: How realistic are herbal remedies? Why follow the path of herbal remedies? and What expectations can you have when it comes to healing with herbal remedies?

Chapter One

Natural Health Through Healing Herbs—An Essential Primer

To begin any discussion about natural health, we need to start with the elephant in the room—legitimacy. This chapter will discuss a multitude of traditional healing practices and how they translate to the modern day. Before being able to discuss anything with legitimacy or defend any claims, we must look at the complicated circumstances that bring us here.

Traditional practices have had a downfall in recent generations. This may be attributed to widespread disbelief in older methods as a valid, respectable practice, which in turn caused practitioners to isolate themselves for fear of ostracization. In discussing herbal remedies with any hope of validity, it is crucial to understand how credibility is affected by the varying vocabulary of the many branches of holistic healing. Even labeling the practice itself comes with its own set of impressions. Terms as clearly discredited as "pseudo" or "new age" science, to more covert, discreet words such as "alternative," "integrative" or "complementary" medication leave us with little room to even name ourselves. While the addition of holistic or homeopathic medicines does not discredit nor disregard pharmaceutical and other conventional methods of treatment, advancements in the field on a larger scale are difficult, to say the least.

One of the reasons holistic medicine regained friction is its claim to fame via many celebrities. While some famous claims can be attributed to hopeful delusion or publicity stunts, celebrity is not the (only) root of disbelief in the field. The relationship between wealth/celebrity and "pseudoscience" is usually explained by three reasons: Dreamed-up-money-grabbing endorsements; a patronizing relationship between time, money and status; and gentrification. On the surface, this might seem explanation enough, but if anything, it allows for a wider discussion that looks critically at health practices.

While unethical, unproven claims have dampened the legitimacy of truthful herbal medicines, it is crucial to remain unbiased and analytical when absorbing these claims so that we may slowly regain validity. These attempts are not always delusional or ill-intended. There tend to be cycling trends among these groups. Some practices may emerge with the best intentions, but rather due to preemptive claims about their capacities, or uncorrelated success, they can fall out of style just as quickly. In these cases, keeping an open mind to new discoveries is not foolish, but extensive research is needed to prove these claims., In addition, critical thinking should be applied to the motivation behind sudden, too-good-to-be-true miracles.

People are realizing that western medicine is not a fix-all and that jumping blindly into using the medication can do more harm than good. It is important to exercise caution when using celebrity-endorsed medications because of these reasons. And yet, taking advantage of the time and money they spent on researching alternative health strategies is not pointless. There is something to be said about celebrities from Kim Kardashian to Richard Gere to Ellen DeGeneres—people with access to unending resources and who practice one form of alternative medicine or another (acupuncture, meditation, traditional medicine, and so on). They illustrate an understanding that there is more to healing than simply western medicine.

Conspiracy and long-winded connections to provable, scholarly research have further created doubt and legitimate concerns about conventional medicine. The understanding of medicine and its short- and long-term effects on a variety of patients in *both* pharmaceutical and holistic fields is ever-growing. Distrust in the medical field is based on intersectional discrimination from test trials to doctors' offices. Privatization of health resources has enabled greed-filled corporations to push more expensive alternatives, regardless of the side effects.

This is not to advocate for complete distrust in conventional medicine. Quite the contrary; it's an explanation of why people end up looking for alternatives. There is reason to treat both herbal and pharmaceutical cures with caution. Disregarding people who look beyond conventional medicine, for whatever reason, is at the very least unempathetic. Beyond that, there are those who may not have access to or success with conventional cures, who deserve relief or see these things as part of their culture. There is room for all these experiences to exist together, and a possibility for health to be something obtainable for all.

For most of history, what we now call herbal, holistic, or alternative medicine was the only form of medicine throughout the world. There is a huge variety based on geography, overlapping with what was available and what values people held. Taking just a quick look at a very surface level description of some of the varieties of traditional medicine, we have traditional Chinese medicine, which includes acupuncture, diet, herbal therapy, meditation, physical exercise and massage; African traditional medicine which consists of divination, spiritualism, and herbalism; and traditional European medicine, which consists of diet, herbalism, spirituality, and superstition. While today we can extend and explain these practices more, this is what kept the human race alive up until very recently. The concentration on strictly "western" medicine has left behind some of the crucial pieces of medicine, the ones that don't view illness in a vacuum.

One of the most obvious connections between the pharmaceutical and the holistic approach is the slow burn reintroduction of marijuana into mainstream society. There was a time, not so long ago, when cannabis was synonymous in many households with any other hard drug. Since that time, we have seen the identity of tobacco in cigarettes become the villain as the long-term effects have been better studied. Cannabis emerged with its faults, but many positive influences as well. While this is not to say it is for everyone, and it is still illegal in many parts of the United States, cannabis has been prescribed as medicine. Studies have found it has been able to help overall (chronic) pain, increase appetite, reduce anxiety, epilepsy, muscle spasms, HIV/Aids, and so on (Jackson et al, 2017). While studies are not conclusive on each of the ailments cannabis has been used for, in general, it has been able to bring an overall sense of well-being to those who are otherwise suffering, physically or mentally. In none of these cases does it claim to be a cure, but for those who are without an affordable long-term solution, the legalization (and therefore safe consumption) of cannabis has been a win. The same is true for those looking for more diverse access to healthcare.

In its wake, another natural medicine has emerged as well. Hallucinogenic mushrooms containing psilocybin have made their way onto the medicinal plant platform. Studies are now showing the possible benefits of micro-dosing mushrooms for a multitude of complicated mental health problems. This research is not fresh either. In fact, Johns Hopkins Research has released research that mushrooms have been proven to treat depression and even Alzheimer's with few side effects (Johnson et al, 2008). There is a fear that the association of recreational drugs with medicine and the herbalism community will create a stigma associated with a platform that is already distrusted. The benefit is that people are proving through word of mouth and through respected studies that there are powerful natural substances benefiting their health in serious, tangible ways.

There is now a push to study the long- and short-term effects of these plants and their chemicals so that they can be accurately prescribed by doctors, eventually. This is a bridge that connects the known medicinal chemicals in plants, with the hope that there will be further study and validation of the safe consumption of herbal remedies. Plants that have been long used in herbal medicine traditions might be able to make a redeeming comeback, and the knowledge that has been passed down in communities will be respected in medical fields once again.

How to Support Your Herbalism Lifestyle for the Long Term

One of the leading themes in this book is to highlight the health benefits of the plants themselves, their ingredients, the act of obtaining those plants, and the process of preserving and using these ingredients. The health benefits are not always quantifiable as pharmaceuticals. Like cannabis, other plant-based remedies are often not recommended as a cure, but for relief of symptoms, whether temporary or chronic. Humans, in general, love to create patterns in things to help understand our world better, and pharmaceutical care does this very well as it reduces the variables and tracks all aspects in charts. This research is luckily how we know they are effective and safe. The downside of this push for understanding and control is when things like herbal therapies cannot be tracked and quantified in ways that are absolute, we cannot make definitive claims about the effects for global use. When we talk about how herbalism can fit into our lives as part of a long-term plan, we need to think of these fluctuations and roadblocks. Herbalism as a lifestyle incorporates more than numbers, but changes how we see health.

There is a multitude of factors that don't fit into quantitative research when it comes to health and medicine. The American Psychological Association has a study that shows being outside helps our mental well-being, even though they say laboratories cannot capture the diverse benefits of time in the outside world (Weir, 2020). So while we know that there *can* be mental benefits from claiming agency to healing in an industrial world, ethically it would be wrong to tell anyone that it *will* work. We might think of herbalism—in part—with regards to the saying, "the whole is greater than the sum of its parts." The reason we do consider *all* of the work involved with herbalism, from learning, to foraging and growing, to creating remedies, is that it becomes who you are, not just what you do. The urge to not rush is because it needs to be organic with your life. It can be a great chore, another thing to do on your list unless you see how it can build and add on to what you already have. When something touches so much of your life and who you are, it is not so simple to say it's only the remedies working.

Joining herbalism means deliberate, conscious, and intentional choices. When you take healing into your own hands, you have to take on the job of many. You need to be more observant and make well-researched choices. It can be very difficult to be self-reflective enough to make these observations and choices. While one person might find a calling in the exertion, it might repel and exhaust another practitioner. One may find the routine of a morning herbal tea is something that sets them up for productive success in the day, while others may find it taxing to add another thing to do in their day. The addition of a hobby for someone who is productive might cause a sense of pride. Others would see it as another job, not tie their self-worth to their ability to produce. Your journey might look different from others because of this. If something is not adding to your life in some way, you should find what works for you.

There are many aspects of the healing journey, and it takes a lot of work to specialize in a healing regimen that works for you and yours. If you simplify this section, it comes down to two main points: Our health can't always be quantifiable, and it is personal and individual, but this is missing a key piece... This personal work requires a great deal of honesty with yourself. To be intentional and observant, you need to be honest about the results you see in your healing, and also with the expectations you have. Being healthy looks different for everyone, and if you are already on this journey, you might have started healing other unhealthy pieces of your life as well. Health can be affected by our entire lives, habits, relationships, work, sleep, exercise, food as well as herbal remedies and so on. All of these things should be included in your healing in a way that works for you.

When we think about long-term change, and how much work goes into it, we might think in reference to diet culture and how much failure is involved. That industry relies on people wanting quick results with little work. Willful ignorance of your own health and habits means you will look at herbal medicine for a miracle cure, and that will only work against you. Time outside, or laughter, can't be prescribed in exact numbers, but the only way to attempt holistic medicine is to see your life as a whole. You are not just pieces existing separately. Be observant of what you need, deliberately choose a path clear of bias and excuses, and begin to h eal.

A Careful Approach

Starting from the outside looking in, it might seem like there is an endless number of plants to learn before you can even get started. If you have picked up this book, most likely you live in New England, which means starting with plants relevant to your location can help refine this load before you even start. With globalization, you are likely to see gardens full of plants from around the world as well. In the wild, you are likely to see more native species, but also taken into consideration in this book is that exotic/foreign plants have become a part of the natural landscape.

As your inventory grows, it will feel like less of an impossible task. Once you start knowing plants as individual species, seeing the differences, similarities, and characteristics of each, adding to this list will be second nature. For example, you might not know a certain plant, but you might know that the mint family is responsible for square stems. You might also notice its smell and texture, narrowing it down through a multitude of options.

If I have learned anything from nature and the path of herbal remedies, it's to be humble. Herbal safety is always the first thing to consider before attempting anything. There exists a lot of misinformation, and extensive research is a sign of a good herbalist. Herbal remedies are not meant to be used the same way as conventional medication and **herbs can and will interact with prescription/over-the-counter medication**. There needs to be a balance of confidence in the field, as well as caution. I have not stopped learning, and if you continue in the field, neither will you. Don't worry about finishing. Once you start, just keep putting one foot in front of the other.

Herbal/plant-based remedies start with raw materials. Many people prefer to forage or grow their own plants to have an assurance of quality and organic status. Some also find mental or spiritual relief in both activities. There is nothing wrong with choosing to buy store-bought herbs, though. In recent years, affordable dry and fresh herbs have been easier to come by. Foraging and gardening are usually interesting to people based on being cost-effective. If by preference, or due to time or physical restraints you choose store-bought herbs, do not feel deterred from continuing on with herbal-based remedies. If possible, farmers' markets and locally sourced grocery stores are a great compromise. If you still like the drying and processing part, you can buy fresh herbs and continue as recommended.

A good way to view herbal remedies is by comparing the benefits of many foods. Most people have heard of the saying "you are what you eat" when it comes to explaining why it's important to eat healthy food. For example, eating a banana is known to be a great snack. It is full of nutrients like potassium that we need to be healthy. But like all things, it should be eaten in moderation. According to the BBC, eating more than seven bananas in a sitting can cause dangerous amounts of potassium (Rhodes, 2015). This is not to mention you would probably end up constipated and so full of bananas you would have less room for other food, causing a nutrient imbalance. Herbs have nutrients in them that can help with easing everyday discomforts, but being reasonable about consumption is just as important as being reasonable about expected results.

Being aware of the dangers of herbal remedies doesn't mean you can't be excited about the many possibilities as well. If cautions about the herbal medicine industry, realistic expectations of treatments, or any preliminary warnings are surprising, uncomfortable, or disappointing, it means they did their job. Herbal remedies, like pharmaceuticals, are not magical, they are not perfect.

Herbs have regained popularity in the last twenty years or so, but they have been around as long as humans have walked the earth. Plant-based medicine is a valid form of knowledge that is important for a well-rounded, medically treated person. Now that we know what to expect from this topic, in Chapter 2, we will start to get to know the plants around us.

Chapter Two

Chapter 2: Profiles of Medicinal Plants in New England

This chapter is about the herbs (including a go-to herbal dictionary) that are available for foraging, cultivating, or obtaining in New England. Chapter 6 will go over foraging in more depth, but we will start off this chapter by introducing beginners to some of the things to expect in the field. Identification is something that most people will never fully master. There are just so many plants. If you spend a lot of your time identifying plants in your area, though, you will become very familiar with the local varieties. This will mean that when there is a plant that you don't know, you will be more aware. Why is this foreign plant here? Why have you not seen it before? This happened to me personally in the last few years with garlic mustard. I had not encountered it for a long time and one day it popped up in my garden. Suddenly, out of nowhere, I started to notice it everywhere (it is an edible invasive species). And so, one more plant was added to my inventory.

One of the problems with exclusively foraging is that there are a lot of exotic and highly regarded herbs that are not available in your area or even the entire USA. Ordering certain herbs online is not always cost-effective and, depending on your reason for connecting to local environments, cannot support your practice. Despite these problems, if you live in New England, there are plenty of medicinal herbs native to the region. Locally sourcing your herbs can give agency to the practitioner, and create a more sustainable practice—plus, even better, they are easily obtainable. Luckily, starting with a local area keeps this knowledge specific, and you won't be worrying about learning irrelevant information. Expanding this knowledge might happen later.

Identification Process

When it comes to identifying a plant, there are some things that might seem obvious to start with, such as whether it is a tree or some sort of herbaceous plant, but there are many other things about a plant's appearance that can help identify it. There are also plant identification apps, but in my experience, they are not totally reliable, and if it is something you plan on eating or healing with, you want to be sure. If it is a plant you have kept an eye on for a while, you might have noticed if it comes back every year in the same spot, or if it may have reseeded, but on the trail, this might not be applicable.

A great place to start identification is ... the place. Location is a huge factor in identifying plants. Of course, reading this book, the location is already set out for you as New England. This will help narrow it down a little bit, especially if you are working with a perennial. Perennial means that it comes back every year. If plants do not die in the winter, you will be able to narrow down which sort of plants are able to withstand that hardiness zone. Hardiness zones are a way of identifying the climate in certain areas for planting. New England consists of zones 5-6, which is also important to know if you are a gardener. The location also refers to the more specific landscape of the plant's environment. Whether the soil is sandy, swampy, in direct sunlight, or on a rocky landscape will all help determine a plant's identity.

When it comes to appearance, the time of year should be taken into consideration. Some plants have different harvest times, and those times won't always be when it's most identifiable. Flowers and fruit are often the most noticeable parts of a plant and can tell you a lot about it. Carefully observe the color, the number of petals or fruit, if there are clusters of flowers, the texture of the petals or fruit, etc. If it isn't the right time of year for the plant to have flowers or fruit, or if their appearance is not helping you narrow down the plant's identity far enough, there are still plenty of characteristics to observe that can help you to identify it correctly. Notice the bark or stem color, texture, width, shape, and height. Is there sap on it anywhere? What do the leaves look like (once again, shape, color, texture, and size)? How do they grow from the plant?

Misidentification

Even those who have extensive knowledge of their local and exotic plants need a refresher. When I was just starting, I remember wanting to know more about a plant in the garden my parents called a "gardenia." While they were accurate with most of their information, this plant was not in fact a gardenia. A gardenia resembles a rose for reference, and the plant in question was around the size and shape of a daisy, with three-point petals that started as red on the inside and were rimmed with bright yellow. I discovered this plant, commonly called many things such as "blanket flower," "Indian blanket," and "Firewheel," is part of the Asteraceae family. Its scientific name is "Gaillardia pulchella," which is where I am sure the information was scrambled—"Gaillardia" and "gardenia" are not so far apart. The point is that there is never a time we stop learning in life, or in this field.

Another great example of identity confusion can come from another field in nature—birds. The bird known in America as the "robin" and the bird in England known as the "robin" are two completely different birds. This did not happen by accident; the birds look quite different, besides their rusty-colored chests, but it was the settler's way of giving a nod to a token of home. Frustratingly, this happens in the plant world all the time as well. Misidentification can happen when there are lots of variants in a plant classification division, like the above-mentioned Asteraceae family, which includes all varieties, from sunflowers to daisies. Misidentification might be also due to confusing names such as plants referred to as the "false" of another plant. The Canada mayflower (Maianthemum canadense) is sometimes referred to as the "false lily of the valley," because of its very similar appearance, but is not related to the real "lily of the valley" (Convallaria majalis). This is by far not the only plant referred to as such: "false spirea," "false Solomon's seal," "false aralia," etc.

Mistaken Identity: Invasive Plants and their Native Look-alikes, an Identification Guide for the Mid-Atlantic (Sarver et al., Nov. 2008), illustrates this point further, comparing native plants with their foreign (and often invasive) look-alikes. These look-alikes might be obviously different enough to avoid disastrous mishaps when it comes to consumption; the invasive "tree of heaven" and native "staghorn sumac" for example. The fuzzy red berries associated with the staghorn sumac are usually the ingredient harvested from the bush and do not appear on its invasive look-alike. This issue might become more problematic, though, if someone were foraging in a season without this obvious characteristic, looking over the other differences (strong odor, milky sap, leaf shape), and transplanting the tree of heaven to their garden. This plant can cause other problems, like releasing a chemical into the soil that can disrupt the growth of other plants. Even if these plants are harmless to us personally, we should beware of encouraging them to grow, even in our own gardens. No matter how careful we are, the wild, from birds to wind, can pick up seeds and pollen that can damage the land for native species. In addition to its look-alike, staghorn sumac also fights for its reputation against "poison sumac" which can give a rash similar to poison ivy, to which it is also related. To identify the poison sumac, you might notice white waxy berries, its wetland habitat instead of dry like the staghorn, the smooth-edged leaves (don't touch), as well as smooth bark, as opposed to the staghorn's hairy branches and berries.

Some misidentified plants go further than damaging the ecosystem and can damage your personal health. Wild grapes and their evil twin, Menispermum canadense, or "Canadian moonseed," can not only be dangerous but *deadly*. The fruit has different shaped seeds (round—grape; crescent—moonseed), taste, and the vine on the moonseed doesn't have forked tendrils like the grape, according to Janet Burns (2016). True versus false morels, wild carrot versus hemlock, wild blueberries versus tutsan berries, and wild tomatoes versus nightshade also made that list.

All of this being said, even a beginner forager should not run into serious problems with misidentification. Being aware of your environment, and taking your time before harvesting, eating, or touching plants you are unfamiliar with, is part of being respectful of your environment, which is step one. Going out and observing plants, taking notes, and asking questions will make you feel a lot more comfortable and capable of identifying correctly. Realistically, as a beginner, you shouldn't begin harvesting until you know, with one hundred percent accuracy, what you are harvesting, what it does, and how much you can take. A plant might even be delicious, but it may be illegal to harvest due to conservation laws. [See chapter 6 for more about the conservation of New England plants.] A lot of the plants that we will talk about in herbal remedies are easily identifiable. The many plants and some of the unique challenges that come from foraging are part of the fun. If you are uncomfortable with foraging one plant because of its risks, there are always many more alternatives instead. Now, let's look at some plants.

Identification and New England Plant Dictionary

This section is formatted for easy accessibility in identifying plants and packs in much useful information for quick referencing. The information selected for each plant contains the most relevant things you need to know in reference to foraging, gardening, identifying, conservation, further research, and of course, medicinal purposes. Plants are organized by type of plant, which will usually be the most notable factor. This categorization is the scientific category. If you cannot find a plant in the section you are looking at, you might find it in another section; some small trees might appear as a shrub, for example.

Woody - Trees

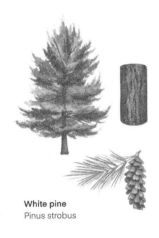

White pine
Pinus strobus

White Pine (Pinus strobus)

Description: Up to 60 feet tall. A fairly straight tree. Dark grayish brown bark that is thick and textured. The needles are green, thin, 2–4 inches long, and look feathery. The pine cone is long, not compact.

Parts used and uses: Young needles are used for sore throat and vitamin C. Poultice of bark can be used for skin healing or for decongestion. Resin is used for respiratory issues, antiseptic, and healing.

Harvest and best form: Bark, sap, and young needles are all harvested in the spring. The bark should be dried. Sap can be used hard or soft. Needles should be used fresh.

Growing conditions: Grows in woods with well-drained soil.

Category: Sweet, bitter

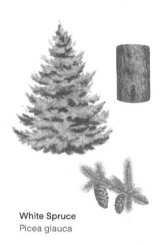

White Spruce
Picea glauca

White Spruce (Picea glauca)

Description: Up to 50 - 130 feet. A fairly narrow tree with thin and scaly bark. The tree has 2-4 in long, rhombic in cross-section, blue-green needles. The cones are hanging, thin and cylindrical.

Parts used and uses: Anti-bacterial, anti-fungus. Cones are used for urinary issues. The inner bark is chewed for viral infections or to create a poultice to prevent infection. Stems and needles are used for tea or bath aroma.

Harvest and best form: Bark and young needles are harvested in the spring. The bark should be dried. Needles should be used fresh. Cones can be harvested in the late summer before they open. Let them dry and release the seeds, then eat fresh.

Growing conditions: Lives in woods with well-drained soil

Category: Sour, sweet

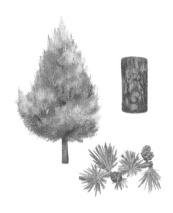

American Larch (Tamarack)
Larix laricina

American Larch (Tamarack) (Larix laricina)

Description: Short, up to 30 feet. Flat and short needles, that are dark green and soft-looking, are lost in autumn and turn bright orange. Very small pinecones that when juvenile are bright red. As a needle tree, it has a typical triangle shape.

Parts used and uses: Bark, flesh, roots, infections, boost immune systems, upset stomach, colds.

Growing conditions: Likes wetlands

Harvest and best form: Can be harvested any time of the year. Best if bark, needles and root are dried before use.

Category: Bitter, sweet

Dangers: May disrupt any immune medicines

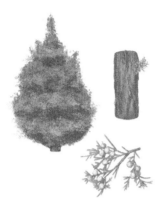

Red Eastern Cedar
Juniperus Virginiana

Red Eastern Cedar (Juniperus virginiana)

Description: Shorter, but up to 50 feet. This tree is common in landscaping because its tightly packed foliage is used for privacy. Flat, scaly, dusty green needles, light reddish-brown, paper, peeling bark. Round to a point foliage/branch. Branches can angle upwards to increase its dense look. Fruit is hard, bluish, small, and round.

Parts used and Uses: Fruits, leaves, colds, lung health, cough

Harvest and best form: Fruits can be harvested in late summer when they are deep bluish purple. Happens every few years. Can be used fresh or dried. Leaves can be harvested any time of year, fresh or dried.

Growing conditions: Harsh soil, pasture-like

Category: Sweet, woody

Danger: Toxic

Black Willow (Salix nigra)

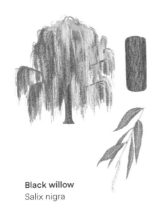
Black willow
Salix nigra

Description: Black willow trees are more compact, with their leaves tighter instead of hanging. Many willow trees have the same aspirin properties, the black willow being just one example, and the one native to the area. The leaves are thin and smooth, and dusty green, but glossy and part of a greater leaflet. The bark is light brown and textured but peeling.

Parts used and uses: Willows are best known for their painkilling abilities, for which the dried bark can be used internally or externally. The leaves can be used for fever. Used in replacement of aspirin.

Harvest and best form: Best harvested in the very early spring. Can be used fresh or dried.

Growing conditions: All willows like very wet areas. Flowers in April. The bark is taken in summer and dried.

Category: Bitter

Dangers: Contains salicin

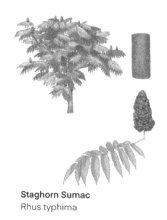
Staghorn Sumac
Rhus typhima

Staghorn Sumac (Rhus typhina)

Description: Up to 20 feet. Leaflets with long, smooth but jagged leaves. Fruit spikes are made of small, tightly packed, fuzzy red berries. Can be a tree or shrub. Leaves are bright red in the fall.

Parts used and uses: Fuzzy fruit is used as an herb in cooking, or to make lemonade. The fruit is used to treat sore throats, improve appetite, astringent, upset stomachs, and for diarrhea. Roots and sap are used to treat boils or warts. The whole plant can be used as an astringent.

Harvest and best form: Harvest fruit in late summer and dry. The root should be harvested in the fall and dried.

Growing conditions: Grows near brush, more likely on hills, or higher land. Flowers mid-summer.

Category: Sour

Mimosa (Albizia julibrissin)

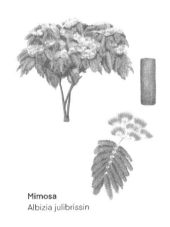
Mimosa
Albizia julibrissin

Description: Up to 30 feet. This tree is tropical-looking. It is smaller, and with a thin trunk, it branches out with smooth, light brown bark. The leaves are fern-like, leaflets that droop long thin, scalloped leaves. The flowers are fluffy-looking, long, white to pink, that fan out in a flat semicircle.

Parts used and uses: Flowers and the bark of the stems are used to treat insomnia and topical infection.

Harvest and best form: Bark is harvested in the spring and dried. Flowers bloom in the summer and should be cooked.

Growing conditions: Likes very sunny places, and only goes as far north as Boston. Likes water, and blooms in the summer.

Category: Aromatic

Peach (Prunus persica)

Description: Up to 20 feet tall. Light reddish-brown bark. Smooth glossy leaves. Papery pink blossoms. Round fuzzy fruit, that is yellow with orange when ripe.

Parts used and uses: Fruit, leaf (early summer), fever, headache, malaria, astringent, relieving constipation, parasiticide, cough, and skin healing.

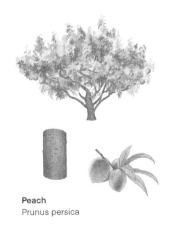
Peach
Prunus persica

The most common use of fruit is to treat bad breath. Full of vitamin C.

Harvest and best form: The fruit is ready later in summer, and the leaves are ready in early summer. They are best used fresh.

Growing conditions: Full sun, well-drained soil. Flowers in April.

Category: Bitter, sweet, sour

Black (Rum) Cherry (Prunus serotina)

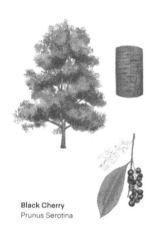

Black Cherry
Prunus Serotina

Description: Up to 60 feet. Long, dark green, and glossy leaves, they turn a bright red in the fall. Peeling gray to rough, red bark. Fruit is dark red cherry-like fruit. The fruit hangs in large groups like grapes. Flowers are small white, 5 petals, and star shaped with feathery stigma, which can be shown in the spring.

Parts used and uses: Root bark is used for aroma and sedative. The bark can be extremely poisonous, and while it can be helpful in very small doses, it's best to avoid ingesting it. Can be infused in cool water as a wash.

Harvest and best form: You can harvest the young and old bark, but young is preferable. Should be dried.

Growing conditions: Likes moisture and fertilized soil. Blooms in late spring. Harvest bark in fall, and store only for one year.

Category: Sweet, sour, bitter

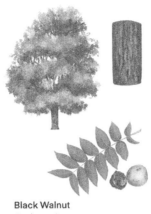

Black Walnut
Juglans nigra

Black Walnut (Juglans nigra)

Description: Up to 120 feet tall. This tree has long leaflets with long, slightly thin green leaves, with hairy undersides. Round fruit starting October that starts off as a green ball the size of a golf ball; inside is the typical walnut. When mature, it can have a very wide trunk and branches with thick, rough, gray-brown bark.

Parts used and uses: The outer shell of the nut is used for parasitic infections.

Harvest and best form: The nuts are ready in the fall. The hulls can be dried, then ground.

Growing conditions: Dense woods.

Category: Pungent, earthy, bitter, sweet

Dangers: Touch dermatitis

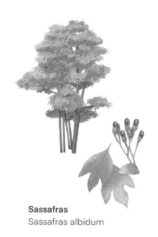

Sassafras
Sassafras albidum

Sassafras (Sassafras albidum)

Description: Up to 82 feet. The green leaves are rounded with three points, but they are bright red in autumn. The flowers are yellow with 6 petals, resembling a daffodil, with thinner petals. The fruit is on long, bright red stems, but the berries themselves are almost black, and the size of a cherry. The bark is thick, "cracked" and grayish brown.

Parts used and uses: The roots and bark are used for digestion, especially anti-parasitic, as a stimulant, urinary tract issues, swelling, skin issues, arthritis, and as an antiseptic.

Harvest and best form: Bark can be used dried or fresh, and is best harvested in the winter.

Growing conditions: Blossoms May-June. Likes well-draining soil.

Category: Sweet

Oak (Red and White) (Quercus rubra), (Quercus alba)

Description: Very tall trees, red oak has smooth, dark bark. Leaves are long, large jagged, with 7 prongs, red prongs are pointed, white is rounded, and not jagged and light bark.

Parts used and uses: Bark is used to treat diarrhea, astringent, sore throats, soothe rashes and burns.

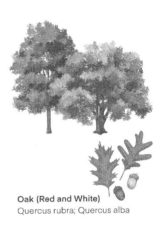

Oak (Red and White)
Quercus rubra; Quercus alba

Harvest and best form: Tree bark is harvested in the spring, then dried.

Growing conditions: Common in the forest, drier climate.

Category: Pungent

Dangers: Medical ingredient tannin can be toxic

Sweetgum (Liquidambar styraciflua)

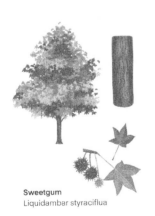

Sweetgum
Liquidambar styraciflua

Description: Up to 82 feet. Thick, cracked-looking grayish bark. Green, smooth, slightly jagged, 5-pointed leaf. The flower looks like a spike of stacked balls of fuzzy stigmas that are tinged red. 1-inch nuts are very spiked.

Parts used and uses: The main part of this tree that's used is the resin. It can be chewed for everything from a sore throat to asthma. It can be applied to the skin for worms, rashes, etc.

Harvest and best form: The resin is best harvested in the late winter and early spring when the sap is flowing. It should be dried before use.

Growing conditions: Likes swampy conditions. Flowers in May.

Category: Pungent

Striped Maple (Moosewood) (Acer pensylvanicum)

Description: Up to 15 feet. The tree is smaller, with smooth green bark. Three-point, jagged, yellow-green leaf. Typically a bright yellow in the fall. The seeds are typical maple samaras, which are commonly known for their spinning with 2 wings that meet in a seed each.

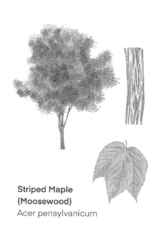
Striped Maple (Moosewood)
Acer pensylvanicum

Parts used and uses: Bark, colds, anti-inflammatory, healing.

Harvest and best form: Best harvested and used fresh in late winter when the sap is flowing.

Growing conditions: Common in forests.

Category: Sweet

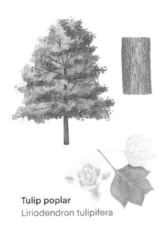

Tulip poplar
Liriodendron tulipifera

Tulip Poplar (Liriodendron tulipifera)

Description: Up to 100 feet. The flower on this tree looks like a tulip, like its namesake. It has 6 petals with a prominent feathery stigma. Their flowers are pale yellow and orange. The leaves in this tree are smooth and round with 4 points. The bark is light brown and heavily striated, giving the appearance of thin stripes.

Parts used and uses: Bark is used as an aphrodisiac, for the wellness of the heart. A tea is made from the bark or roots as a diuretic, for cold and flu symptoms, or to clean wounds.

Harvest and best form: Tree bark is harvested in the spring and dried.

Growing conditions: Likes moisture. Blooms in early summer.

Category: Sweet and astringent

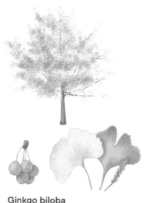

Ginkgo biloba

Ginkgo (Ginkgo biloba)

Description: A taller tree, up to 120 feet. Branches are free forming. A young tree is sparse and slender, as it matures, the tree becomes thick and more lush. The bark is light brown and rough. The leaves are fan or triangle-shaped, but the slender point is at the base of the leaf, and it has a broad, flat, (slightly rounded) end. They are also lobed or scalloped on the end, but smooth edged on the side. Yellow in the fall.

Parts used and uses: The leaves are the part mostly used for cognitive issues such as memory, illness like Alzheimer's, and mental health issues like depression.

Harvest and best form: The leaves are picked in late summer and can be used fresh or dry.

Growing conditions: Full sun, well-draining soil

Category: Bitter

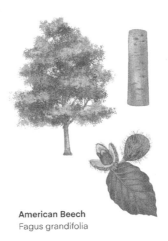

American Beech
Fagus grandifolia

American Beech (Fagus grandifolia)

Description: Up to 50-70 feet tall. White/ gray, paper-like bark and very thick lower branches. The nuts have long spikes oblong and orange. Leaves are oval to a point, slightly jagged with prominent veining, and a glossy dark green to pale orange in autumn.

Parts used and uses: Leaves: Skin conditions (such as poison ivy), headache relief. Inner bark: Improve digestion, may cause abortion, Nut/seed: Roasted for energy, extracted oil for hair.

Harvest and best form: Leaves are best in the spring when they are young, and should be used fresh. Nuts are ready in late summer, best roasted. The inner bark can be harvested when the tree is young. Tea is made from fresh bark.

Growing conditions: Needs rich, well-watered, well-drained soil. Dislikes pollution or salt (avoids roads).

Category: Bitter

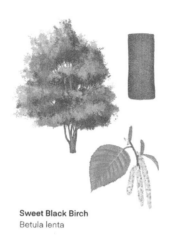

Sweet Black Birch
Betula lenta

Sweet (or Black) Birch (Betula lenta)

Description: Up to 50–70 feet. Simple, green, jagged leaves that turn yellow/orange in the autumn. When young, it has smooth, gray bark that peels to show a reddish brown. When mature the tree might get a thick cracked-looking gray bark. Long, caterpillar-like hanging flowers.

Parts used and uses: Bark, fever, stomach, anti-inflammatory, bladder infection, gout.

Harvest and best form: Harvested any time of the year. Should be roasted and ground.

Growing conditions: Dense forest, East Coast

Category: Sweet, cooling

Danger: Toxic

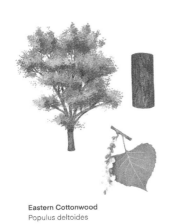

Eastern Cottonwood
Populus deltoides

Eastern Cottonwood (Populus deltoides)

Description: Up to 50 feet. The tree has fewer branches but is very thick. Typically a mushroom shape. Thick, hard, deep indented, grayish bark. Small heart-shaped jagged leaves (yellow-green to yellow in autumn). Seeds are cotton-like.

Parts used and uses: Bark, scurvy, pain relief, fever, anti-inflammatory, cold treatment, encourages healing topically.

Harvest and best form: Bark is typically harvested in the spring, and dried.

Growing conditions: Found in swamps

Category: Bitter

Mulberry (Morus Alba)

Description: Very short tree or shrub. Thick, rough gray bark. Fruit is like long blackberries, red when not ripe, oval, light green, and medium jagged leaves.

Parts used and uses: Berries are used to lower cholesterol, iron, vitamin C, and antioxidants.

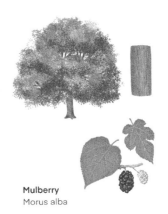

Mulberry
Morus alba

Growing conditions: Does well near the coast, found in brush with dry, poor soil conditions.

Harvest and best form: The fruit is best used fresh. They can be harvested throughout the summer.

Category: Sweet, sour

Danger: Unripe berries cause nausea and possibly hallucinations. and all parts contain latex.

Linden (Basswood) (Tilia americana)

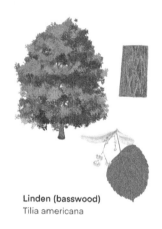

Linden (basswood)
Tilia americana

Description: Up to 60-80 feet tall, this tree can look fairly large. Thick, rough, gray bark. Dark green, and watery, heart-shaped, jagged leaves. Small yellow flowers early to mid-summer, and in the fall the leaves typically turn yellow/orange. From a distance, the tree can look triangular, coming to a point at the top, and the branches spreading wide lower to the ground.

Parts used and uses: Flowers, leaves. All cold symptoms, headache, fever, calming, sleep, bladder control, lung health, boils.

Harvest and best form: Flowers appear early to mid-summer and are best used fresh.

Growing conditions: Dense forest

Category: Sweet, sour

Dangers: Medicinal, beware of consumption

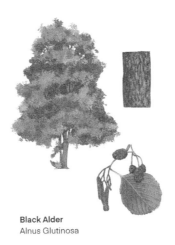

Black Alder
Alnus Glutinosa

Black Alder (Alnus glutinosa)

Description: 60–90 feet tall. Smooth greenish bark. The silhouette changes, but when tall has a long oval shaped foliage, that only leaves 6–10 feet of the branchless trunk at the bottom. Heart-shaped, green leaves that can look glossy. Long, thin, green seed pods that at maturity look like small, round, green then brown pinecones.

Parts used and uses: Dried bark and leaves are used for soothing a sore throat, relieving constipation, fever and swelling, astringent, and healing scabs.

Harvest and best form: Harvest bark and leaves in the spring. The leaves are best used fresh, the bark must be dried before use.

Growing conditions: Likes damp areas. Not fussy.

Category: Bitter

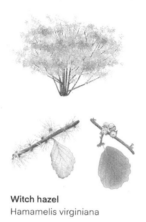

Witch hazel
Hamamelis virginiana

Witch Hazel (Hamamelis virginiana)

Description: Up to 16 feet. Can also be a shrub. The bark of this tree is shiny and smooth, with a dark red tone on new growth. On the trunk, it is light brown and smooth. The leaves are a pale yellow-green that is rounded with deep veins. The flower is noticeable by its pink center but with long, string-like petals that are pale yellow.

Parts used and uses: The bark is used for swelling, pain, skin irritation and as an astringent. The leaves are used for inflammation and hemorrhoids. Internally the bark is used for menstrual issues and diarrhea.

Harvest and best form: Harvested in the spring or fall. Can be used dry or fresh.

Growing conditions: Blooms in the late fall. Likes wooded areas but needs enough sun.

Category: Bitter, astringent

Woody - Bushes/Shrubs

American Spikenard (Aralia racemosa)

Description: Up to 6 feet. This shrub is flatter-looking, with large, round, teardrop leaves that are slightly textured. It gets a large spike of dropping, semi-transparent, rich berries, like small grapes.

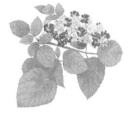

Parts used and uses: The root is what is mainly used in medicine as a stimulant, for coughing, induces sweating, and helps joint pain. Externally it is used for eczema and other skin conditions.

American spikenard
Aralia racemosa

Harvest and best form: Root is taken in late summer and dried.

Growing conditions: Thick brush. Blooms in early summer.

Category: Sweet

Hawthorn (Crataegus monogyna)

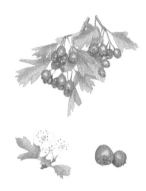

Hawthorn
Crataegus monogyna

Description: Up to 20 feet. Leaves have 1 spike on either side and a scalloped flat end. The berries are bright red and hard. Small, white florets, in a star shape, with stigma ended with a red point. Light brown bark, slightly cracked, but thick.

Parts used and uses: The main use is for heart conditions from strengthening the heart to spasms, but both the fruit and the flowers are also used as a sedative. The bark is used for malaria.

Harvest and best form: Harvest fruit in the fall. Best used fresh.

Growing conditions: Blooms late spring. It likes woods and brush.

Category: Sweet and sour

Guelder-Rose or Cramp Bark (Viburnum opulus)

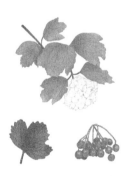

Guelder-Rose (Cramp Bark)
Viburnum opulus

Description: Up to 16 feet. The leaves have 3 points and are jagged. They are watery and green. The berries are bright red on long stems. The flowers are white, star-shaped, in a spiked floret.

Parts used and uses: The bark is used for reducing spasms, specifically in digestion or for menstrual use. Leaves are used for constipation and inducing vomiting.

Harvest and best form: Bark is best harvested in spring or fall. Best used dried and ground.

Growing conditions: Blooms early summer. Likes damp woodland.

Category: Pungent

Cranberry (Viburnum trilobum)

Description: Up to 10 feet. Gray bark. The flowers are white in a flat floret. 3-point, jagged, watery leaves. Bright red cherry-like berries.

Parts used and uses: Bark and roots have been used to treat uterine collapse. Roots induce vomiting.

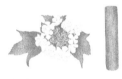

Cranberry
Viburnum trilobum

Harvest and best form: Bark and root can be harvested in spring. Best used dried.

Growing conditions: Blooms late spring. Moist, lowlands.

Category: Sour

Spicebush (Lindera benzoin)

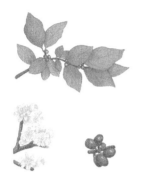

Spicebush
Lindera benzoin

Description: Up to 9 feet. The leaves are simple, smooth, and green. In the fall, it is bright yellow. Blueberry-like, bright red berries. Green blooms with feathery stigma. Smooth brownish bark.

Parts used and uses: Bark and twigs are used to induce sweating, for colds and muscle pain, and the bark especially is used for intestinal worms.

Harvest and best form: Harvest twigs and bark in spring, use dried.

Growing conditions: Likes moisture, likes wetlands. Blooms in the spring.

Category: Warm

Prickly Ash (Zanthoxylum americanum)

Description: Up to 13 feet tall. 2-inch thorns cover the bark and can be a small tree. Smoothish, green/brown/red bark. Round, cherry-like fruit in clusters. Small white florets. Leaflets of round, thick, smooth, and long leaves, that slightly curve inward.

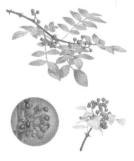

Prickly ash
Zanthoxylum americanum

Parts used and uses: Bark and fruit are used for menstrual cramps, oral health, and induce sweating and circulation. The fruit is also used as a stimulant and for digestion. Fruit is numbing topically.

Harvest and best form: Fruits in summer, best used dried.

Growing conditions: Blooms late spring. Likes dry and rocky ground.

Category: Astringent, sweet

Dog Rose (Rosa canina)

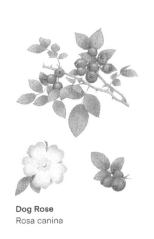

Dog Rose
Rosa canina

Description: Up to 4 feet. This shrub might climb, or tilt over. Smooth light green or reddish-brown stems, covered with thorns. Thin, smooth, oval leaves. Loose flowers, unlike traditional roses, open completely in a star pattern. Typically, light pink to white. Rosehips replace flowers if only petals were picked. Hard red-ish berries, full of seeds.

Parts used and uses: The fruit is used for joint pain, the immune system, sore throats, as a diuretic and laxative. Used topically for skin health.

Harvest and best form: Flowers in summer, fruit in fall, used fresh or dried.

Growing conditions: Likes sandy, shrubby areas. Blooms early summer.

Category: Bitter, sweet, aromatic

Partridgeberry (Mitchella repens)

Description: Ground crawler, 5 inches tall. Smooth, red, woody stem. Oval, smooth, thick, glossy leaves. Cherry-like fruit. 4 petals, white flower.

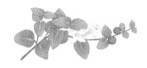

Parts used and uses: Leaves are used to induce labor. Helps with sleeping and is a diuretic. Externally can be used on hives. Berries are a sedative.

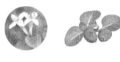

Partridgeberry
Mitchella repens

Harvest and best form: Harvest leaves in summer, best used dried. Berries late fall to summer.

Growing conditions: Blooms early summer. It likes dry woods. Berries mature in late fall

Category: Sour

Barberry (Berberis)

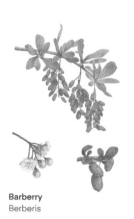

Barberry
Berberis

Common barberry (B. Vulgaris), cultivation of this is prohibited in Connecticut, Massachusetts, Michigan, and New Hampshire due to rust fungus. The Japanese barberry (Berberis thunbergii) is invasive in 32 states, and a common place for ticks. **Toxic to Dogs. Thorns may be poisonous. Not all barberries are edible.**

Description: Deciduous shrub, 3-14 feet tall. The leaves are toothed, ovate, alternate, pale green outside and grayish beneath, and yellow flowers.

Parts used and uses: Stems, root, bark: Used as yellow dye. Berries: Vitamin C, berberine (also found in goldenseal), relieve diarrhea, fever, stomach, improve appetite and well-being.

Harvest and best form: Best used fresh, harvest in fall.

Growing conditions: Most barberries grow in zone 4–8. Full sun–partial shade. Loamy, well drained 6–7.5 pH. Not super fussy.

Category: Sour

Blackberry (Rubus fruticosus)

Description: Up to 9 feet. The bush can be vine lined with thorns. Older stems are reddish. The leaves are lightly textured, jagged, and green. The fruit is thick and solid, unlike a raspberry, and can be more elongated. Red when young, black when ripe. White/pink flowers, 4 petals with feathery sigma.

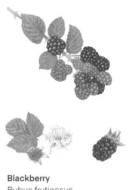

Blackberry
Rubus fruticosus

Parts used and uses: The root can be made into a gargle for mouth issues. It's an astringent and diuretic. Used for digestive issues.

Harvest and best form: Root harvested in fall, best used dried.

Growing conditions: Adaptive. Blooms all season.

Category: Sour, sweet

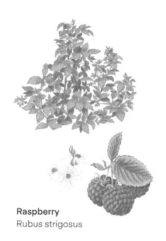

Raspberry
Rubus strigosus

Raspberry (Rubus strigosus)

Description: Up to 6 feet. The red stem of this plant is covered in thorns, right up to the fruit. The leaves are heart-shaped and textured, with slightly jagged edges. The fruit on the plant is a soft, hollow berry that's bright red. The flower is small, a white star shape.

Parts used and uses: Leaves and roots are used for anti-inflammatory, decongesting, to induce childbirth, for menstrual issues, and as a stimulant. Can be used for oral health and on wounds for healing.

Harvest and best form: Leaves are harvested in late summer and dried. Root harvested in fall, best used dried.

Growing conditions: Blooms through summer. It likes dry brush areas.

Category: Sweet and sour

Japanese Knotweed (Reynoutria japonica)

Description: Up to 9 feet. Small white florets, spikes. Large, round, dark green, oval-point leaves. Dusty red, smooth bark.

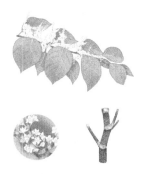

Japanese Knotweed
Reynoutria japonica

Parts used and uses: The root is used in treating lung conditions, mouth conditions, skin issues and as a diuretic. The leaves can also be used for treating skin conditions.

Harvest and best form: The root is harvested in fall. Best used fresh.

Growing conditions: Blooms all summer. Likes wet lowlands.

Category: Sour

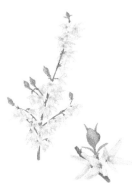

Forsythia (Lian Qiao)
Forsythia suspensa

Lian Qiao (Forsythia suspensa)

Description: Up to 16 feet tall. Smooth, green, thin oval leaves. The bark is smooth and reddish. The shrub is covered in weeping, bright yellow flowers from every branch.

Parts used and uses: The flowers are antibacterial; a poultice is made for skin issues. The fruit is used for treating airway issues, as a stimulant and topically for pain.

Harvest and best form: Flowers in spring, fruits in summer, best used fresh.

Growing conditions: Blooms in spring. Prefers grassy areas or on slopes.

Category: Mild

Sweetfern (Comptonia peregrina)

Description: Up to 5 feet. A low-lying green fern. Round scalloped edges. It is technically a shrub, but looks like a fern with a thicker stem. Fuzzy green flowers.

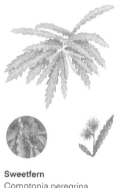

Sweetfern
Comptonia peregrina

Parts used and uses: The leaves are used mainly for digestive issues, specifically Crohn's disease. Externally used for skin ailments, especially rash from the poison ivy family.

Harvest and best form: The leaves are harvested in summer and best used fresh.

Growing conditions: Likes sandy, dry places.

Category: Bitter

Black Elder (Sambucus nigra)

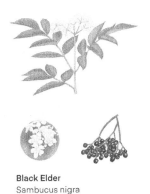

Black Elder
Sambucus nigra

Description: Up to 20 feet. Small geometric stems at the end of branches have small white flowers. The fruit is very dark and grape-like. The bark is gray and papery.

Parts used and uses: Young stems and flowers are used for skin wounds. The fruit can be used as a laxative. Flowers are used for coughing, inducing sweating, as a stimulant and astringent. Leaves are used topically for pain. Older bark and leaves can induce vomiting when eaten.

Harvest and best form: Young stems picked in spring. Flowers in summer. Best used dried. Fruits in late summer - do not eat raw

Growing conditions: Likes fertile soil, lots of sun.

Category: Sweet, aromatic, bitter

Wild Sarsaparilla (Aralia nudicaulis)

Description: Typically no more than 1 foot, but crawls across the ground. Smooth, simple leaves with deep veining, but with small teeth that form on leaflets. Flowers are a sparse-looking, global shape, with feathery stigma on long stems. Dark, blueberry-like fruit, on a global floret.

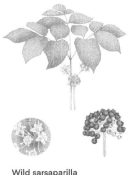

Wild sarsaparilla
Aralia nudicaulis

Parts used and uses: The root and the leaves are topically used for a variety of skin conditions. The root is collected in autumn. They are both also considered a stimulant and can be used for common cold and flu symptoms like coughing, and stomach aches.

Harvest and best form: Harvest roots in fall. Best used fresh.

Growing conditions: Likes a shady, moist area. Blooms in late spring.

Category: Sweet, Pungent

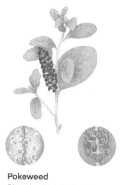
Pokeweed
Phytolacca americana
(herbaceus)

Pokeweed (Phytolacca americana) (herbaceous)

Description: Up to 6 feet. Bright red, smooth stem. Berries are very dark on long spikes, drooping towards the ground. The leaves are yellow green, smooth and oval pointed. Flowers are small, unnoticeable white and fleshy on the spike.

Parts used and uses: Use with caution, this plant contains narcotics. The root is used to treat rheumatism, skin issues, and pain. It is also an anti-inflammatory and is used for fever. The fruit is used topically for sore breasts and as a tea for rheumatism.

Harvest and best form: Harvest root in autumn, fruit in summer. Best used fresh.

Growing conditions: Flowers late august. It likes damp and rich soil.

Category: Neutral, bitter

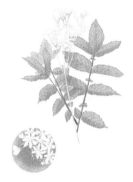

Meadowsweet
Filipendula ulmaria

Meadowsweet (Filipendula ulmaria)

Description: 4 feet tall. Spirea is like a bush. Floret spikes or white flowers with noticeable fluffy/ feathery stigma. 3-point, dark green, textured leaves. Dark red, smooth bark.

Parts used and uses: Flowers are used as painkillers (aspirin), for diarrhea, and heartburn. Dried for scent. The root topically can be used for sores. Leaves and stems are used as antiseptic, astringent and to settle the stomach.

Harvest and best form: Flowers in summer, best used dried.

Growing conditions: Likes swamps and wet areas.

Category: Bitter

Comfrey (Symphytum officinale)

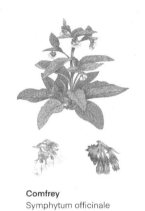

Comfrey
Symphytum officinale

Description: 4 feet tall. The stem is green and fuzzy. The leaves are long and thin, and green but textured. The flowers are long trumpet-shaped florets of dark pink.

Parts used and uses: The roots are used. Externally used for healing the skin. Used topically for back pain.

Harvest and best form: Fresh or dried, best harvested in fall.

Growing conditions: Likes moisture and shade. Flowers in the spring.

Category: Neutral

Wintergreen (Gaultheria procumbens)

Description: Less than 1 foot. Thick, glossy leaves, simple, long. The leaves are dark green to dark red. Bright red cherry-like berries. This plant likes to cover the ground. White flowers will hang from the stem.

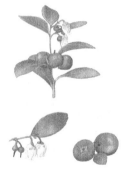

Wintergreen
Gaultheria procumbens

Parts used and uses: The leaves are used for pain (aspirin); anti-inflammatory, stimulant, and used externally for pain.

Harvest and best form: Young leaves and dried.

Growing conditions: Acidic soil. Blooms mid-summer.

Category: Cold

Periwinkle (Vinca minor)

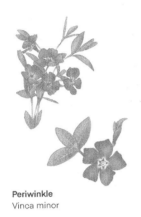
Periwinkle
Vinca minor

Description: Up to 1 foot. Ground crawler, but dense. Thick, glossy, dark green, oval leaves. 5-petal purple-blue flowers.

Parts used and uses: The leaves are used for several bleeding issues such as menstruation, wounds, as well as oral health and as a sedative. Roots are used for low blood pressure. T

Harvest and best form: Leaves are evergreen. The root is harvested in autumn. Best used dried.

Growing conditions: Likes moisture; wet areas or wooded areas. Blooms late spring.

Category: Cold

Woody-Liana (Woody Vines)

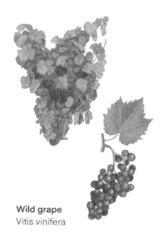

Wild grape
Vitis vinifera

Wild Grape (Vitis vinifera)

Description: Up to 50 feet. The vines of this plant can suffocate even trees. It has a larger main stem and smaller tendrils that wrap and clip. The leaves are wide and jagged; the fruit is a green or purple berry in a loose triangle spike.

Parts used and uses: Unripe fruit is used for sore throats and as a laxative. The ripe fruit is used as a diuretic, to cool, for strengthening veins, and as a laxative. The leaves are used for bleeding and calming the stomach.

Harvest and best form: Best used fresh, fruit is ripe in fall.

Growing conditions: Likes moisture, blooms late spring.

Category: Mild and sweet

Japanese Honeysuckle (Lonicera japonica)

Description: Up to 16 feet. Small, round, but long leaves. They are dark green and glossy. The bark is light brown, but peeling, long strips. The flowers are yellow and white, and the 2 petals open. Dark, smooth berries.

Japanese honeysuckle
Lonicera japonica

Parts used and uses: The flowers are antibacterial, antispasmodic, and anti-inflammatory, aid in pain, digestion, and cold symptoms. Externally, the flowers are used for rashes. Harvest in the morning.

Harvest and best form: Flowers in spring to early summer, best used fresh.

Growing conditions: Likes rich mountain earth.

Category: Sweet

English Ivy (Hedera helix)

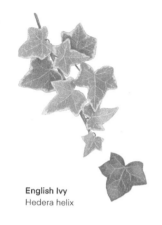

English Ivy
Hedera helix

Description: Up to 50 feet. A climbing vine, with 5-point shiny leaves.

Parts used and uses: This plant is toxic, so consumption is not recommended. The twigs can be used on burns. The leaves are anti-bacterial, anti-fungal, and anti-parasitic.

Harvest and best form: Twigs harvested in spring, leaves in summer, both best used dried.

Growing conditions: Loves to climb, prefers shade. Flowers in the fall.

Category: Bitter

Ground Ivy (Glechoma hederacea)

Description: Less than 1 foot tall. Round, scalloped leaves with a slight texture. Small iris-like purple flowers. Minty taste.

Parts used and uses: Used to treat mucus issues. Leaves are used for fever, appetite, painkillers, worms, energy, and digestion. Can help with bruising.

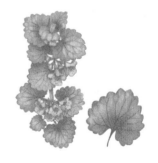

Ground Ivy
Glechoma Hederacea

Harvest and best form: Harvest in summer, use dried or fresh.

Growing conditions: Likes damp, wooded areas. Blooms in spring.

Category: Strong, cold

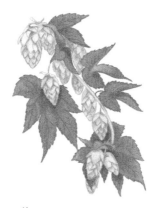

Hops
Humulus Lupulus

Hops (Humulus lupulus)

Description: Up to 20 feet. The fruit that comes off the plant is pale green in a pine cone-like shape and is what is considered the "hops." The vine is thick, but not technically woody. The leaves are long, teardrop-shaped, jagged, and textured. Citrus, pine tasting.

Parts used and uses: The fruit of the hops plant is used for many, many ailments like cough, fever, insomnia, boils, nerves, worms, and more. The flowers are also used for swelling and uterus issues. Aromatherapy for pine and earthy smells.

Harvest and best form: Fruits are harvested from late summer to autumn, use fresh or dry.

Growing conditions: Sunny, woody areas. Flowers mid-summer.

Category: Astringent, pungent

Herbaceous – Graminoids (Grasses)

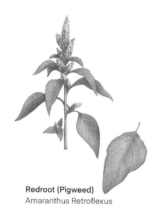

Redroot (Pigweed)
Amaranthus Retroflexus

Redroot/Pigweed (Amaranthus retroflexus)

Description: Up to 2 feet. Can be a shrub. Thick stem and textured, jagged leaf. Red to pink root. Seed spike at the top of the stem. Annual.

Parts used and uses: The leaves used for tea make an astringent, for menstrual and other internal pain, digestion and sore throat. Caution for high nitrates.

Harvest and best form: Harvest all summer, best used fresh or dry.

Growing conditions: Common weed. Harvest all summer.

Category: Astringent, neutral

Wild lettuce (Lactuca virosa)

Description: Grows as tall as 6 feet. Green, long, very jagged leaves. Looks like a dandelion with a tall, thick stem.

Parts used and uses: Sap can be used as a painkiller, narcotic, digestive, and sedative. Infusion of the plant leaves can be used to treat insomnia.

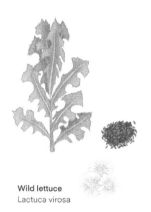
Wild lettuce
Lactuca virosa

Harvest and best form: Leaves and sap harvested spring through summer, best used fresh.

Growing conditions: Common weed, especially in grassy areas.

Category: Mild, pungent, bitter, sweet

Cattails (Typha latifolia)

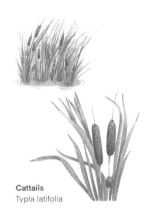
Cattails
Typla latifolia

Description: Grows as tall as 8 feet. Bright yellow-green, thin, coarse leaves. Soft brown catkin up to 1 foot long. Perennial. Warning—Look-alike: Iris Plant. Identification: All leaves come from the ground.

Parts used and uses: Do not use if pregnant. Burned leaves are used as a topical antiseptic and internal diuretic. Fresh ground roots are used on all topical issues. The sap is used as an antiseptic and for toothaches. Pollen is used to increase menstrual flow, is superlative, and encourages healing. Cattails can be used as a form of cotton for poultices or bandages.

Harvest and best form: Harvest in the fall. The pollen is dried and the roots fresh ground. Sap in summer use fresh

Growing conditions: Grows in shallow water. Find mid-summer.

Category: Sweet and bitter

Danger: Don't use if pregnant

Sweet Flag (Acorus calamus)

Description: Grows as tall as 6.5 feet. Bright yellow-green, thin, coarse leaves. Long, spike seed pod. Iris-like yellow or purple flowers. Perennial.

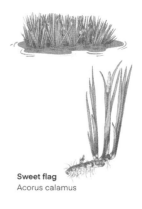

Sweet flag
Acorus calamus

Parts used and uses: Young leaves raw or cooked used for sweetness. Roots in their second or third year are used for digestion, stimulation, and pain, and to increase appetite. May be toxic to eat and cause miscarriage. Used as an insecticide, as a spray or as incense. May be used for aromatherapy. The dried root can be stored but has a short shelf life.

Harvest and best form: Roots in their second or third year in the fall and used fresh. Young leaves use raw. Harvested in autumn.

Growing conditions: Grows in shallow water. May to July. Look in place with cattails, like ditches and water banks.

Category: Sweet to bitter, with warmth

Herbaceous - Forb (Flowering)

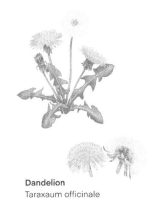

Dandelion
Taraxaum officinale

Dandelion (Taraxaum officinale)

Description: Up to 1 foot. There are many species of dandelion, but this is the most common. Dandelions are well known, dark yellow, stringy petal flowers. When they go to seed, they have a cotton-like, global head. The stems are pink and green, succulent-like and hollow. The leaves are long and typically lie on the ground. They are long, green, and textured, with many deep points, and jagged.

Parts used and uses: The whole plant is used. Used for liver health and antioxidant, as well as a diuretic and laxative. Can be used for energy.

Harvest and best form: Leaves and flowers are harvested in spring and summer, roots in the fall. Best used fresh or dry.

Growing conditions: Dandelions are a common weed and grow in most places, but prefer open areas.

Category: Bitter, pungent

Coltsfoot (Tussilago farfara)

Description: Up to a foot tall. This plant is commonly misidentified as a dandelion, as it has dense, stringy, yellow petals. This plant, when opened, has a flatter look like a daisy though, with a darker yellow center. The leaves are round but pointed and scalloped all around, light green in a small centralized pile, and have small teeth on the stem.

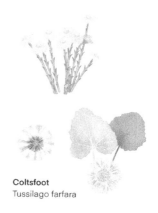

Coltsfoot
Tussilago farfara

Parts used and uses: The flower is used for any infection of the respiratory system.

Harvest and best form: Blooms very early spring to mid-spring. Use fresh or dried.

Growing conditions: Likes moisture and is a common weed in unfertile soils.

Category: Bitter

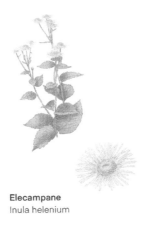

Elecampane
Inula helenium

Elecampane (Inula helenium)

Description: Up to 5 feet. Another dandelion look-alike. This plant is part of the daisy family and looks more similar to coltsfoot. This plant has less stringy petals and a center that is flat and less hairy. The leaves are large and climb up the stem and look quite dense. They are slightly textured, long, and smooth rimmed.

Parts used and uses: The whole plant is used, especially the root. The most common use is for lung issues. Also used as a sedative, immune booster, and digestive. Use topically for bacteria and fungus.

Harvest and best form: Harvest root in fall, the rest in the summer. Best used fresh or dry.

Growing conditions: Likes moisture and is found with other dense weed areas in the shade. Blooms in the summer.

Category: Pungent

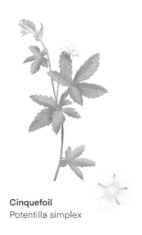

Cinquefoil
Potentilla simplex

Cinquefoil (Potentilla simplex)

Description: Up to 4 inches. Cinquefoils might be mistaken for buttercups, as they have small, yellow, star-shaped flowers, but buttercups are poisonous when fresh. The cinquefoils have long red stems, and leaflets that are sprouted from a center point to create a circle. The leaves are glossy and jagged. Can seem vine-like.

Parts used and uses: The plant's roots are used for an oral health gargle.

Harvest and best form: Harvest root in the spring, best used fresh or dry.

Growing conditions: Sometimes a weed likes open, dry areas. This flower indicates poor soil. Blooms in the summer.

Category: Pungent, astringent

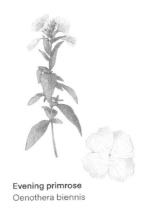

Evening primrose
Oenothera biennis

Evening Primrose (Oenothera biennis)

Description: Up to 5 feet. The leaves are long and pointed, and tight to the plant, so they curve upwards. The leaves are shorter at the top, giving the plant a triangular look. The blooms are about 2 inches and a pale yellow. They open in the evening at the top of a spike.

Parts used and uses: Leaves and flowers are used for relaxing, intestinal, and menstrual issues, especially symptoms of premenstrual syndrome.

Harvest and best form: Harvest all parts in the summer. Best used dried.

Growing conditions: Likes sandy, weedy, and sparse areas. Blooms in the summer.

Category: Pungent

Agrimony (Agrimonia eupatoria)

Description: Up to 2 feet tall. Bright yellow flower spike with noticeable perky stigma. 5 petals in star formation. Seed pods resemble green burrs. Light green textured, jagged, elongated oval to a pointed leaf.

Parts used and uses: The whole plant is used as a digestive aid, for jaundice,

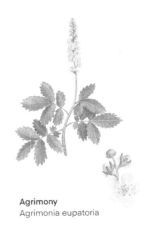

Agrimony
Agrimonia eupatoria

sore throat, and as an astringent. Used for external healing.

Harvest and best form: Harvested from late spring to mid-summer. Can be dried.

Growing conditions: Grown in thin soil cover, with other weeds, full sun.

Category: Bitter, sweet, dry

Mullein (Verbascum densiflorum)

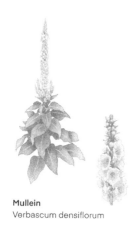

Mullein
Verbascum densiflorum

Description: Up to 4 feet. The mullein plant is sometimes referred to as nature's toilet paper because it is soft and fuzzy, and used by campers. It is pale green. Leaves go up the stem and at the top are long spike florets. The flowers on the mullein plant are yellow and give the plant a weedy look.

Parts used and uses: The flowers and leaves are used to treat a large variety of ailments that affect the respiratory system, depression, and headaches. Topically treats sores.

Harvest and best form: Harvest in summer, use dried.

Growing conditions: Likes dry, meadow-like areas, but not fertile soil. Blooms in the summer.

Category: Mild, pungentu

Sweet Clover (Melilotus officinalis)

Description: Up to 4 feet. The plant starts off looking like a simple clover. There are three leaves, but these are slightly more oval-shaped, and solid green. It gets taller and has long, thin branches with florets that are yellow and weedy.

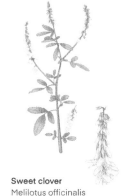
Sweet clover
Melilotus officinalis

Parts used and uses: It is used as a diuretic and to treat poor circulation. The flowering plant is used for cramps, varicose veins, and insomnia. Externally used for swelling.

Harvest and best form: Harvest in summer, use dried or fresh.

Growing conditions: Likes grass, most likely part of the lawn. Blooms in summer.

Category: Bitter

St. John's Wort (Hypericum perforatum)

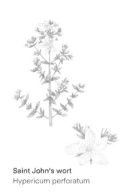
Saint John's wort
Hypericum perforatum

Description: Up to 2 feet. This plant can look like a shrub. With thin stems that send out two thin, elongated, cool green leaves in rows. The flowers are yellow, star-shaped, with a feathered stigma center.

Parts used and uses: Most used for treating depression, can boost immunity and encourage healing. The flowers and leaves are used.

Harvest and best form: Harvest in summer, use dried.

Growing conditions: Blooms late spring to summer. Likes drier areas with slight cover.

Category: Bitter

Goldenrod (Solidago virgaurea)

Description: Up to 2 feet. Goldenrod is often mistakenly blamed for seasonal allergies when the true culprit is ragweed. The plant is a thin, sometimes drooping plant with small, thin, and elongated leaves. The foliage is light green and clips the stem in an alternating pattern. At the top is a head of yellow, drooping florets of very small flowers.

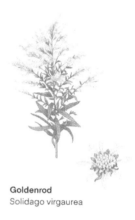

Goldenrod
Solidago virgaurea

Parts used and uses: Leaves and flowers are used. Used for thrush and urinary tract infections. Used topically for its healing and blood clotting, it is antiseptic and anti-inflammatory.

Harvest and best form: Harvest all parts in the spring and summer. Best used fresh or dried.

Growing conditions: Common weed found in ditches and other non-desirable places. Likes drier areas. Flowers from spring to fall.

Category: Bitter, astringent, hot

Black-eyed Susan (Rudbeckia hirta)

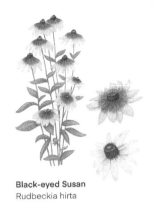
Black-eyed Susan
Rudbeckia hirta

Description: Up to 2 feet tall. Thin, green, hairy stems. Few small, thin, smooth leaves. 4-inch-wide. Bloom, with bright yellow, thin long leaves. Domed-shaped, black or brown center. Perennial.

Parts used and uses: The root infusion is used for worms, snake bites, earaches, and colds.

Harvest and best form: The roots are harvested in the fall and best used fresh.

Growing conditions: Loosened soil. Summer to autumn.

Category: Astringent, sweet

Sunflower (Helianthus annuus)

Description: Up to 9 feet. Sunflowers are a huge family. This one has a standard look with a very large bloom, looking like a daisy. The petals are large and yellow, with a large, brown center. Sunflowers have a thick, green, fuzzy stem. The leaves are tear dropped and jagged edged.

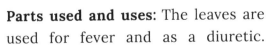
Sunflower
Helianthus annuus

Parts used and uses: The leaves are used for fever and as a diuretic. Topically can be used on bites or sore skin. The petals are used for malaria and lung ailments. The roots are used as a soak for pain.

Harvest and best form: Harvest leaves and petals in summer, root in fall, use dried or fresh.

Growing conditions: Likes dry, sunny places. Blooms in the summer.

Category: Pungent

Beggarticks (Bidens frondosa)

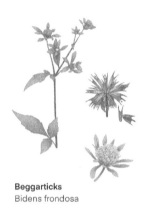

Beggarticks
Bidens frondosa

Description: Up to 5 feet tall. 1, maybe 2 or 3 bright yellow-orange flowers, like an unbloomed dandelion. Light green textured, jagged, long, feather-like, hairy leaves. Thick, red woody stem. Dark brown seed heads.

Parts used and uses: The root is used in a tincture for irritation, urinary tract issues, inflammation, and pain.

Harvest and best form: The root is harvested in the fall. Best used fresh.

Growing conditions: Likes lots of moisture and sun.

Category: Neutral to bitter

Borage (Boraginaceae officinalis)

Description: Up to 2 feet. 5 triangle shaped petals in a blue/purple color or white. 4 long prominent fuzzy sepals in between each petal. Long, thin, but coarse leaves that fan around the plant, are used as a salad leaves. The leaves and the stem are covered in soft fuzz and are light green.

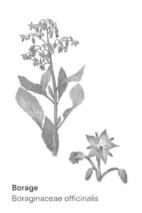

Borage
Boraginaceae officinalis

Parts used and uses: Flowers and leaves are used to boost joint restoration, healthful skin, and increase immunity.

Harvest and best form: Bloom in summer. Best used fresh or dry.

Growing conditions: Likes less fertile ground and blooms all summer. The flower lasts longer if the dead blooms are removed to encourage more growth.

Category: Bitter, mild

Chicory (Cichorium intybus)

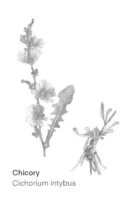

Chicory
Cichorium intybus

Description: Up to 5 feet. The chicory plant is best identified by its pretty blue-purple flower. It has long, overlapping petals, like a daisy, but a less prominent, small, white center. The flower is attached right to the long stems. The petals are flat and scalloped on the ends. The plant itself is not used as an ornament as much because it is long and spindly without much foliage, besides at the bottom. These spindly branches sprout from the ground with dandelion-like leaves.

Parts used and uses: The most common use of this plant is a coffee made from the roots. It also suppresses appetite and digestion. The rest of the plant can help with an upset stomach.

Harvest and best form: Harvest root in autumn.

Growing conditions: Commonly found in open grassy areas, or ditches. Blooms from summer to fall.

Category: Bitter, pungent

Jewelweed (Impatiens capensis)

Description: Up to 4 feet. The most noticeable part of the jewelweed is the flower that droops slightly. It comes in a range of colors. It has 3 petals in a trumpet-like shape. These flowers stick up above the dark green, simple flowers on the stem by a long, bare stem.

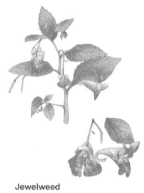

Jewelweed
Impatiens capensis

Parts used and uses: The leaves are used for treating skin issues, mainly poison ivy rash.

Harvest and best form: Harvest in the spring and summer. Best used fresh.

Growing conditions: Moist, lowland woods. Flowers from summer to fall.

Category: Sweet, pungent

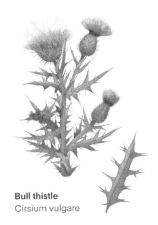
Bull thistle
Cirsium vulgare

Bull Thistle (Cirsium vulgare)

Description: Up to 6 feet. This plant is well known as a sharp, annoying weed because it's covered in thorns. Its flower is a stringy purple, cotton-ball-like, on top of a thorny green bulbous base. The flower turns into a cotton-like seed head, like a dandelion. The stem is reddish. Leaves are long, with spine-like, jagged points, like dandelions, but thinner and covered in spikes.

Parts used and uses: The roots and leaves are used for stiff muscles and nerves. Leaves can be used as diuretics.

Harvest and best form: Roots are harvested in the fall, leaves in the spring, and are best used fresh or cooked.

Growing conditions: Common weed, prefers open over woods.

Category: Mild

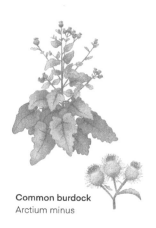
Common burdock
Arctium minus

Common Burdock (Arctium minus)

Description: Up to 4 feet. Common burdock and bull thistle might be confused for each other because of the flower. The flower on the burdock is also purple and stringy, but much smaller, only just sprouting out of the bulbous base. The base is also less like spikes but with little hooks. Dried, this is the plant that annoyingly attaches to clothes. It is also adorned with a smooth stem, and simple green, veined leaves.

Parts used and uses: Root is used as a detox. The plant itself is antibacterial and antifungal and used to treat skin conditions from acne to ringworm.

Harvest and best form: Root is best used fresh, harvest in fall.

Growing conditions: Common weed, it likes brush. Blooms all summer.

Category: Sweet

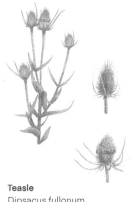

Teasle
Dipsacus fullonum

Teasle (Dipsacus fullonum)

Description: Up to 6 feet. This plant is another one that is similar to the burdock. It is similar due to the spiked head but differs as there are thick spikes that curl up from under the teasle bloom. The bloom itself has small purple flowers but they are more tubular than stringy. The entire plant is covered in thorns. The leaves are long and crumpled. May have multiple branches.

Parts used and uses: The leaves are applied to the skin for healing. The root is said to help digestion and acne.

Harvest and best form: Harvest leaves in summer, root in fall, use fresh.

Growing conditions: Rough, thick soil. Blooms in the summer.

Category: Bitter

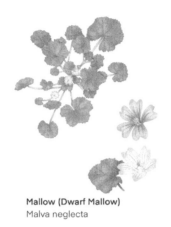

Mallow (Dwarf Mallow)
Malva neglecta

Mallow (Dwarf Mallow) (Malva neglecta)

Description: Up to 2 feet. The mallow plant has a thick, wood-like stem. When it is young, the plant is to the ground, and long herbaceous stems with leaves protrude from a centralized spot. The leaf has 6 faint points but is circular and jagged. The flowers come off the tall stem, and blooms in a usually pinky-white flower. The flower is delicate like a poppy, but larger and more cupped.

Parts used and uses: The leaves and flowers are used externally for swelling and healing. Internally, it is used for the respiratory, urinary, and digestive systems.

Harvest and best form: Harvest in the summer, best used fresh or dry.

Growing conditions: Likes unfertilized and dry areas, and is a common weed in some places. Blooms all summer.

Category: Neutral

Field Garlic (Allium vineale)

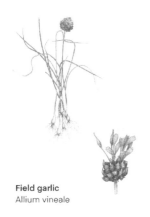

Field garlic
Allium vineale

Description: Up to 2 feet. This plant is grass-like, with long, thin, hollow, dusty green leaves. It grows a stringy petal, purple flower.

Parts used and uses: The whole plant is used for allergies, digestion, hypertension, as a stimulant, and for deworming.

Harvest and best form: Harvest in the spring and summer. Best used fresh.

Growing conditions: Likes dry, grassy areas, blooms in the summer.

Category: Pungent

Garlic Mustard (Alliaria petiolata)

Description: Up to 4 feet tall. This plant is single stemmed and is smooth and green. The leaves coming off the stem are teardrop-shaped and jagged, with texture. The flowers are small, white and star-shaped.

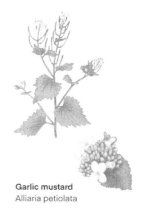

Garlic mustard
Alliaria petiolata

Parts used and uses: Use with caution. Leaves and stems can be used to treat cold symptoms and encourage coughing mucus. Treats fever. Topically used for skin conditions and worms.

Harvest and best form: Harvest in the spring and summer. Best used fresh.

Growing conditions: Blooms in the spring. Invasive in damp, shaded areas.

Category: Bitter

Indian Tobacco (Lobelia inflata)

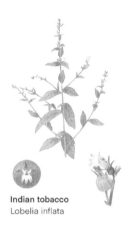
Indian tobacco
Lobelia inflata

Description: Up to 2 feet. A less impressive-looking species of this genus, the plant is tall with alternating leaves up the stem. The leaves are simple and green. At the top bloom the light purple flowers. These flowers are not dense though and only bloom a few at a time.

Parts used and uses: Everything above ground is used, but mostly the leaves. Helps with depression, asthma, other lung conditions, and memory. Can induce vomiting.

Harvest and best form: Harvest all parts in the late summer. Best used fresh or dried.

Growing conditions: Likes dry meadows. Blooms in the summer.

Category: Sweet

Danger: Overuse of this plant can be fatal. Refer to a professional before using.

Mugwort (Artemisia vulgaris)

Description: Up to 4 feet. Dark green leaves that are feather-like in shape, with jagged edges. It has been veins and an angular reddish-brown stem. The flowers are reddish and fluffy but unattractive. The plant itself is very weedy-looking.

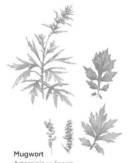

Mugwort
Artemisia vulgaris

Parts used and uses: Leaves can be dried and smoked for relaxation and for dreaming. Used in pain, especially menstrual issues. Helps the nervous system.

Harvest and best form: Harvest in summer, use dried.

Growing conditions: Grows in weedy areas, blooms in the summer.

Category: Bitter

Ragweed (Ambrosia trifida)

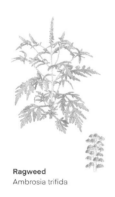

Ragweed
Ambrosia trifida

Description: Up to 6 feet. Ragweed is one of the main seasonal allergens. It is a tall plant that branches out and up into many thin spike florets. The stem is sturdy and red. The leaves are yellow, green, and smooth, with 3 points. This version of ragweed does not have as prominent yellow flowers as some and has very small, ball-like pollen sacs.

Parts used and uses: The leaves can be used on bites. The root is used to treat menstrual pain. Internally, the leaves can be used for fever, cramping and diarrhea.

Harvest and best form: Harvest all parts in summer, and early fall, use dried.

Growing conditions: Common weed, and adaptable. Blooms late summer to fall.

Category: Warm

Shepherd's Purse (Capsella bursa-pastoris)

Description: Up to half a foot tall. Is a single, long-stemmed plant. It has a central leaf blade at the bottom that splays out feather-like leaves on the ground. There are some smooth, longer leaves on the stem. At the top of the plant are straight, thin branches that jut out 1-2 inches with small flowers. The head of the plant has a flat florets head, with white, 4-petal flowers.

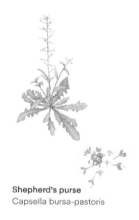

Shepherd's purse
Capsella bursa-pastoris

Parts used and uses: The parts above the ground are used as a clotting agent, for bladder infections, circulation issues, and headaches.

Harvest and best form: Harvest in summer, use dried or fresh.

Growing conditions: The plant is a weed and is adaptive. Likes dry soil.

Category: Warm

Stinging Nettle (Urtica dioica)

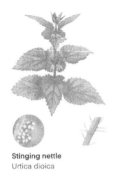
Stinging nettle
Urtica dioica

Description: Up to 4 feet. The stem is red, with a layer of fuzz. The leaves are long triangles with jagged edges that are lined up with the plant. The fruit is a drooping, thin stake of very small, fuzzy pinkish berries. **Causes severe skin rash.**

Parts used and uses: Commonly used for pain. The leaves are also used for anemia. The whole plant is used for heart health, inflammation, and as a clotting agent.

Harvest and best form: Harvest in spring, use dried or fresh.

Growing conditions: An adaptive weed, dislikes acidic soil. Blooms all season.

Category: Neutral, salty

White Horehound (Marrubium vulgare)

Description: Up to 1 foot. The leaves are heart-shaped and highly textured. They are a dusty green color and are scalloped on the edges. The leaves and flowers protrude in rows up the stem. The flowers are small and not notable but in thick ball-like clusters. Tastes minty.

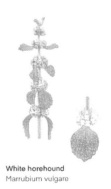
White horehound
Marrubium vulgare

Parts used and uses: The leaves are used for coughing, cold and mucus. It is antiseptic and can help with muscle contractions, energy, and digestion.

Harvest and best form: Harvest in summer. Use dried or fresh.

Growing conditions: Flowers all season. It likes weedy places.

Category: Cold

Yellow Dock (Rumex crispus)

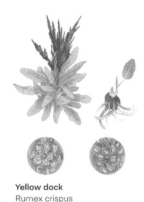

Yellow dock
Rumex crispus

Description: Up to 2 feet. Very long, thin leaves that are lightly curled or wrinkled, grow from one central point in the ground and splay out. The flowers are spike florets with heart-shaped pink, yellow and greenish, open pod-looking flowers.

Parts used and uses: The root can be used internally as a laxative or externally for a range of skin problems.

Harvest and best form: Harvest in spring or fall and use dried.

Growing conditions: Common weed, flowers all season.

Category: Bitter, sour

Herbaceous - Fern

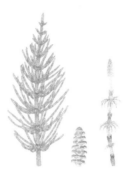

Field Horsetail
Equisetum arvense

Parts used and uses: The parts above the ground are used to clot blood. This can help speed healing time. Good for hair and nails. It has properties for internal use, but without professional dosing, it can be dangerous and not recommended.

Harvest and best form: Harvest in summer and can be dried.

Growing conditions: Invasive, like to be well-watered.

Category: Mild

Chapter Three

Creating Your Own Herbal Remedies Part One: Basic Processes and Techniques

I caution people against going overboard on gathering herbs for plenty of reasons, but one less noble than conservation is the amount of work to process. Being out in the field looking at plants can be a wonderful time, but when you get home, the work doesn't end, it is just beginning.. The process isn't difficult, but it is absolutely necessary. Plants go bad really quickly, so they need to be dealt with right away.

The process with which you will be treating your plants should be considered, ideally, before you harvest. If you are planning to dry the plant, hanging it might be the most convenient way, but you might not be harvesting the whole plant, or the plant might not be the right type for such. Having a plan before harvesting can help with this process so that you can leave enough room. As plants wilt so quickly, limiting the amount you gather will ensure you can start processing everything as quickly as possible.

We are assuming now that your plant(s) are completely identified (foraging and garden herbs are covered in later chapters), but there is a little technique for harvesting as well. Some plants may be harvested at odd times, but for the most part, you can tell when a plant is at its peak in the season. You want to use your senses; if it looks, smells, and feels healthy, it probably is at its most potent. I have the habit sometimes of trying to use the damaged, older part of the plant and leaving the nice-looking stuff behind, but this is a sure-fire way to miss the pieces that are holding the most potential. A tip I first learned about roses and then applied to harvesting aromatic herbs is that picking the plant first thing in the morning is optimal for more flavor. It may help to harvest leaves when the dew on them has evaporated to enhance the drying process. Finding the perfect time might be impossible, but take these tips into consideration. Depending on the plant, you may opt to remove only the petals, leaving the flower head, or maybe only taking a few leaves.

Drying and Garbling Medicinal Plants

Drying

Drying is often the way to go when it comes to preserving plants. It is a great way to preserve potency, but this varies according to the herb and how it is stored. On average, herbs can be stored for up to two years at their highest potency. The interesting part about dried herbs, though, is that their "best before" date does not mean they will spoil. Unless herbs are very old, "expired" herbs will not be unusable, just milder in flavor and medicinal benefits. The drying process doesn't take much, but there are some key things to consider.

The simplest way to dry is to bind the plant or a bundle of the plants/plant parts with some sort of string. If the plant is dense or heavy, make sure not to over-pack them. You want to make sure that the plant is able to dry completely, which cannot happen if water is trapped in between the plants. As some plants dry, the stems will shrink with water loss; I make sure this binding is tight enough to accommodate this. Your plant might be more difficult to bind if its stem is smooth, or leaves don't cross. The binding string can slip off, so to avoid this, zigzagging the string between the stems as well as binding the outsides can help.

You can then hang these bound plants from a hook, or if you have room, you can hang multiple bundles from a stick. This stick might just be held up between two surfaces or hung on a wall. Whichever way you find is best for you, make sure it is stable and fairly undisturbed. As the plants dry, they will become brittle; if bothered, this can cause a mess and loss of inventory. It's best to keep them in the shade, but in well-ventilated areas of your house. Direct sunlight may degrade their potency, and airflow is important as they are drying, to prevent humidity from causing mold.

Another way to dry herbs might be a drying screen, where the plants are laid out on a screen, without touching, to dry. This alternative takes up more space but can be a little more organized and efficient in drying.

The process and drying part are just part of the fun, but if this is a part you would rather skip, then food dehydrators work to speed the process and reduce mess as well. If you can avoid it, I would, but using your oven to dehydrate plants is also a method of drying. There are a few reasons this isn't the greatest; ovens are often too hot, and the plants end up being cooked or burnt instead of having the moisture in the plant slowly burned off. This leads to a loss of potency. Once when drying roses, I thought of using this method... the result was not exactly pleasant smelling, and the lovely pink color turned an unpleasant yellow. This is not to say oven drying won't work when done right, and herbs often do change appearance and smell when dried. If you don't have the time or are limited to this option, it can work, but the lowest and slowest your oven can go might be the only way it is possible.

Garbling

Garbling means separating the parts of the plants you will and won't use for herbal remedies. The garbling process might be done before or after the drying process. For some plants, it might be necessary to do this before, for a variety of reasons, such as wanting to avoid having the brittle plant break and combining the usable and unusable parts by accident. Either way, it's important to remember that not all parts of the plant are considered equal. Even if all parts of the plant are safe to eat, if a recipe calls for only the heads of a flower, throwing in the whole plant when measuring will dilute whatever benefits the heads specifically have. Refer to chapter 2 to see which parts of the plants you use, but always try to be accurate, even if it's not necessary.

Storing Dried Ingredients

Drying herbs is a step taken to extend the shelf life of herbs way beyond their life as fresh plants. Once this step is done, though, you need to store your herbs correctly to ensure they retain their potency. The storing process is just as important as drying. Just as herbs can be damaged or ruined in the drying process, so can that happen during the storing process. Here is a list of things you should take into consideration as you store your herbs:

- Use airtight containers
- Keep away from direct sunlight
- Keep containers in cool, dry places. If you already have an herb cabinet, that will work
- Make sure to label the name of the herb, the harvest or purchase date, and the day it should be used by (for premade main and plant labels you can go to SilviPavlova.redbubble.com)

Fresh Herbs

There are lots of reasons to preserve herbs for later use, but also many for wanting to use them fresh; the recipe might call for fresh herbs, you like the taste and texture, you might not like any of the preserved methods, etc. There are still some ways that you need to treat your herbs after garbling to make them usable.

- To use the herbs that exhibit maximum freshness, look out for wilting, spots, sliminess, etc.
- Hearty herbs stay fresh longer, leafy herbs spoil quicker. When debating which one to use first, use the one most likely to spoil first
- Keep leafy herbs perky by storing in water and putting them in the fridge, or if storing dry, use a towel to dry as much as possible to prevent mushiness
- Remove store-bought herbs from packaging, trim the stems before storing, wash and treat them with the recommended methods above

Other Methods of Storing and Preserving

In the next chapter, we are going to go over the form of some herbal remedy concoctions. There are a large variety of ways in which you can use these herbs for healing purposes, from taking them internally to using them externally. First, let's talk about some more advanced ways to store herbs as individual ingredients. Some of these methods may be less applicable for using the herbs in remedies later, but can produce ingredients for cooking. Your diet is a great way to start using herbs for healing purposes, whether you're just starting or you're an expert. If you know the form your herbs are going to take from the concoctions listed in Chapter 4, some of these methods might be preferable to others.

Like dried herbs, to keep preserved herbs in their best shape, make sure they are stored properly. All herbs should be kept away from the sun, in cool areas. Keep your containers for these herbs sealed. These are possible medicinal ingredients, so making sure that you treat them as such, to keep out bacteria and mold, is a necessity.

Pickling and Canning Herb Recipe

There are a lot of ways to preserve food. For most of history, people didn't have electricity. When it came to being able to keep food edible throughout the winter, people had to be creative. Some of these methods are more or less preferable. Starting with canning, which has its own varieties, you are able to can anything from meat to fruit. Canning comes with its dangers, though. If you are not experienced in canning and are not able to treat and seal properly, you can waste all of your food. Canning can also lead to botulism poisoning. One of the safer methods of canning is pickling. Pickling is fairly easy, but the downside is that it can reduce the potency or nutritional value, which is especially important when we are talking about herbal use. If you are focusing on any water-soluble nutrients, they might be lost in the pickling process. Pickling herbs might be a great way to preserve herbs for dietary use, but is not useful for topical recipes.

One of the reasons you might choose canning or pickling is if you are looking to start trying herbal remedies by adding them to your diet. Another reason might be that you are comfortable with canning and use this practice in your life already. Herbs can be added seamlessly to your lifestyle this way.

Fermenting

The fermentation of herbs might have additional benefits due to the fermentation process. The most popular example of this is kombucha, a fermented tea. The fermentation process is also used in making yogurt and kimchi. Kombucha can work as a probiotic, as well as provide vitamin B. Probiotics are great for digestion. Kombucha can be made from black or green tea. Of course, green tea is also known for its benefits, such as antioxidants. Kombucha has its faults as well, as it can cause liver issues due to the amount of lactic acid, cause allergic reactions, and can contain alcohol. In addition, there's an increased risk of introducing bacteria and mold when it's being prepared. You can add your herbs to kombucha as you prepare it, as a way of preserving them.

Fermenting might also be done in a separate process, such as in water and salt brine. This process still has lactic acid because it's created in the fermentation process. This can be done with dry herbs as well. Fermenting can also be done in honey. You might choose this way to preserve some herbs if you are interested in storing them for a future prospect of creating a digestion wellness remedy.

Freezing Herbs

Freezing herbs might be the way to go when it comes to cooking or ingesting them. The reason this might be a preferred method for the herbs that freeze well is it might be the closest you can get to fresh herbs. There is more to freezing herbs than throwing them in the freezer, though. The benefit of freezing anything is being able to forget about it until it is needed. The freezer can get hectic, and storing your plants so they are optimal until you use them is really important. There are a few ways to freeze herbs:

1. Some herbs can be stored as-is in an airtight container.
2. Freeze herbs in water. Leafy herbs benefit from this, as ice cubes can be convenient.
3. Freeze in oil, often used for cooking, but topical oil infusions might work as well.

Immersion

Immersion, when it comes to preserving plants, means to "immerse" them into another substance, such as oil, honey (syrup), or alcohol. This might be either the end result of a recipe or an ingredient. It may be something that you are already doing when creating herbal remedies, such as a tincture, but when it comes to preserving, you might do this with fresh or dry herbs as an individual or multiple herb concoctions. Depending on what you are preserving, you can use this oil, alcohol, or honey in external or internal recipes as well. When doing this, whatever substance you are using to preserve will create an infusion, and can/should be used in your remedy or recipe as well to get the full effect.

Salt and Sugar Curing

Salt and sugar have both been used to draw water out of plants and meat. It is a drying method, and the salt and sugar might become an infusion that is used as an ingredient as well or just a tool as part of your processing. Something to be cautious of when it comes to curing with salt and sugar is not over-adding the plants. Unlike immersion, the over-packing of plants may be a problem to a certain extent. You want to make sure in salt and sugar curing that you have enough of the curing agent to draw out the moisture, and eventually dry it, otherwise mold or clumping will be an issue. The choice between salt or sugar is one that can be made based on intended future use or flavor. For example, some sweet flowers such as lilac are used to make lilac sugar. Storing herbs/plants with a complimentary flavor profile means they can be made into an herb-infused salt for recipes.

Using fresh herbs is always a bonus, but it sadly isn't always possible. The methods of preserving in this chapter might be a way for you to add these herbs to your cooking or herbal remedies. Some herbs might be used as-is for whatever treatment you are looking for, some might need a more elaborate recipe or form. How each of these forms takes shape and is used is outlined in detail in the next chapter.

Chapter Four

Creating Your Own Herbal Remedies Part Two: Modes of Preparation

In the previous chapter, there was a lot of information on preserving herbs. The medium in which your remedies are created will have a longer or shorter life span. You might cross-reference how you preserve your herbs with common recipes, to preserve more than one herb together. As an herbalist, you have access to a wide range of methods to prepare herbal remedies for use. There's a reason for each form these remedies take. From targeting specific areas to getting the highest potency, you are taking these ingredients in a fairly basic form and turning them into usable medical ingredients.

This chapter is meant to answer some questions. We have started to break the mysterious walls around this practice, but this chapter takes a look at what format these cures come in. Those who think that herbal healing is potion-making will be able to see the simplicity behind these remedies. In fact, these remedies might start to seem boring once we see that lotions and syrups are not as outrageous as some might expect.

Besides getting a better idea of what the final product of these remedies will look like, this chapter is also about what certain words mean when it comes to herbal medicine, and what the differences are. Every form explained in this chapter might not be referenced in the future chapter on recipes. This nuance is more for a wider understanding of herbal medicine, when the form is referenced. Knowing the vocabulary in herbal medicine is important when it comes to finding reliable information. We need to determine whether using more uncommon words somehow makes their information more valid. As you expand, knowing what kind of "potion" someone is talking about can help you determine if it's reliable or not.

There are, of course, more forms of consuming remedies that are better left for conventional medicines. Whatever form you find best suits your herb therapy needs is up to you. The main way of consuming the herbs not listed in this chapter is eating them as part of a recipe. As I have mentioned a few times throughout this book, if you are able to add herbs with the intention of health upkeep as well as adding flavor to your dishes, you should. This can be thought of as taking your multivitamin for overall health. The remedies in this chapter are targeted for more specific issues that need a strong treatment.

Extract

Extract is the verb, or action of taking something from something; for example, the water *extracts* the taste from the tea. You might see this word used in a different way on shelves like "vanilla extract." In this case, it means the extract of vanilla, but it is actually a tincture, as it takes liquid form in alcohol. Unless you have high-quality processing machines, the extraction of the pure medicinal chemical of a plant is not possible in our home remedies.

Infusion

Infusion is an umbrella term for a substance that sits in liquid to extract its benefits. An infusion might happen in the preserving process as the herbs sit in liquid. It means that the liquid is infused with the herbs and their properties.

Maceration

This is an infusion of finely chopped ingredients. This might mean that it is very strong because the ingredients have been exposed to a higher surface level of liquid and can leach out of a larger area.

Common Herbal Ingredients

You might notice, as you learn about the different ingredients that go into a lot of remedies, that you see a lot of the same things over and over again. As we try to bring a stronger backbone to the herbal therapy community, I think it's important to look at these ingredients as well. Asking "why?" is always a good idea when learning and thinking critically about anything.

Honey

Honey is something that you might see quite commonly in home remedies, for a mixture of scientific and convenience reasons. As long as honey is stored properly, with no addition of water, it will not go bad. Honey has also been proven to have antibacterial, antioxidant, anti-inflammatory properties, and contains a small amount of minerals iron, zinc, and potassium. It can soothe sore throats as well. It can also be a convenient way of making a remedy pleasant to consume. Honey is not a miracle cure. It has these properties but is not meant to replace pharmaceuticals. Not all honey is considered the same; the treatment, source, and purity of honey affect medicinal properties.

Water

Water, like honey, is not all created equal. Whether it's distilled, filtered, well, or city water, its source, and its composition in terms of minerals, greatly affects the water itself. For creating a mixture that is going to be the most shelf-stable, getting distilled water means that it does not have any variables that might complicate your recipe. Water in these recipes serves a variety of purposes. In some, it may be to dilute a concoction, to extract, as well as to hydrate. If someone is sick, they might be losing water in a variety of ways, or even feeling sick due to a lack of water. In these cases, adding some salt and sugar to a glass of water can help replenish electrolytes.

Alcohol

One of the historical uses of alcohol was as a disinfectant in water in Ancient Greece, among other places. It is not recommended to use this as a purification method today, but we still use alcohol as a disinfectant and antiseptic in things such as hand sanitizer. It is used in mouthwash as well. You will see alcohol used in tinctures because it is very effective at extracting useful parts of a plant, as well as keeping it on the shelf longer. Alcohol as an umbrella term usually refers to vodka or brandy, which are 40% alcohol or 80 proof.

Beeswax

Like honey, beeswax comes from bees. There are some studies about the medical properties of ingesting beeswax, but in the form of these herbal remedies, it is usually used as an aid in topicals. It has been used for bruising, inflammation, and burns. Another benefit of using it in herbal remedies is that it is hydrophobic and rarely causes reactions.

Oil

Oil can be a misleading term. Almost all plants can be made into some sort of oil product, though we are not worried about making our own oil here, just using it as an ingredient. The oil that you use will depend on the type of remedy you are creating. The first distinction is edible/ingestible oil and topical oils. There are plenty of oils that you use on your skin and hair, with a plethora of benefits, that should not approach your lips. Because of this, it is hard to give a specific answer on why oil is used in herbal remedies. Oils also all have very different shelf lives and can spoil.

Topically, oil can be used as a carrier, which is a way to dilute essential oils. Essential oils are very strong and can be harsh or irritating on the skin. However, they do have their own variety of benefits. These oils might be used to create a lotion, salve, etc. Oils for the skin include olive oil, coconut oil, jojoba oil, apricot kernel, sweet almond, argan, rosehip, grapeseed, avocado, and more. Each of these oils is composed of different nutrients, and depending on your goals, will all suit you differently. These oils are used topically because of their ability to soak into the skin or moisturize.

Oil for the use of ingestion is a little different. These oils are also used to extract, or as we learned before, preserve. Studies have found that a lot of edible oils such as olive oil, or avocado oil do have antibacterial properties, as most things we eat have some health benefits. Oils for ingesting that are used to extract might also be used as a carrier oil. Infused oils have the potential to cause botulism if not stored carefully.

Glycerin

Glycerin is sometimes used medically as a laxative but is used in a huge variety of skincare products. Glycerin is used as an aid in moisturizing.

Internal

The following forms of remedies are made for internal use. If you are consuming herbal remedies, you are expected to be responsible for what you are taking and making.

Water Infusion

Water infusions are the easiest remedies to make with just water and your fresh or dry herbs. They are made by using hot or cold water to extract herbal properties. This process can take from three minutes to twenty-four hours.

Tea or Tisane

Tea is the simplest way of preparing herbal remedies. While it isn't the only way of preparing and consuming herbal remedies, it is easy and effective—that's why it has been used for centuries. Heat water to the desired temperature. Not all teas are made at the same temperature. Let steep for three to fifteen minutes. Serve as desired. If you see a remedy referred to as a tisane, it just means herbal tea.

Decoction versus Steep

Unlike steeping tea, where water is usually brought to a boil and poured over the tea, this method is used to extract herbal compounds from hard plant parts, like roots and barks. This is done by simmering the plant parts for about thirty minutes. Decoction might be referred to as a tea, as well as an infusion.

Distillation

Refers to collecting the condensation of a boiled liquid to get a more purified version. The benefit of doing this is to remove any plant material and be left with a purified version. This will be a lot more shelf-stable.

This can sound really complicated, but it can be done in your kitchen fairly easily, even without extra equipment. Put a clean brick inside of a large pot and fill the pot with water up to the top of the brick and place a heat-safe container on top. Put your herbs in the water. Put the lid to the pot upside down on the pot (this only works if your lid is domed). Bring water to a light boil, as low as possible as long as it is creating steam. If the temperature is too hot, you might overcook the herbs. Let boil down until you have the desired amount of distilled water. Once in a while you may put ice cubes on the lid to cool it down and encourage condensation.

Tincture

Tinctures are extracts made from soaking and dissolving substances in alcohol. It is essentially infused with alcohol or vinegar. The alcohol used in making a tincture is 80 to 180 proof (40-90%), depending on what type of herb you are using. The plants are cleaned and soaked in this alcohol for at least a month and a half. This process is used to extract a very strong infusion of the medical properties of a plant. The strength comes from the high concentration, but also because the alcohol has already done the job of breaking these chemicals down for use. The benefit, besides the strength, is its form makes it fast-acting as well as having a shelf life of up to five years.

Oxymel versus Electuary versus Infused Honey versus Syrup

Oxymel is a mixture of acid, usually vinegar and honey, to create a tonic or syrup, it is made and taken right away. If it is left to sit, it is a honey tincture. Electuary is a medical (powdered) ingredient plus honey, made and taken right away. Letting it steep would create infused honey. Syrup is created as a thick, sweet vessel for medicine, and is sometimes pure honey.

Powders

It's unlikely an herbal remedy's final form is a powder. You might need to grind herbs into a powder for a remedy, or even a food recipe to increase potency.

Smoke and Inhaling

Herbalism has a plethora of different ways to breathe in herbs. The problem with any inhalants, besides personal effects, is that pets are sensitive to both smoke and essential oils. Smoke can be made from charcoal bricks (typically with resin), incense sticks or cones, inhaling with a pipe, etc. (Note: Indigenous people ask others not to use the term smudging or to use white sage. Celtic practices use the term saining instead). While no studies encourage inhaling smoke, there have been studies to prove some herbs might have benefits. At the very least, inhaling essential oils through a diffuser might be a way of relaxing.

External Preparations

Many of the remedies outlined in the internal section might also be used externally, such as a tincture, any water infusion, and on occasion some electuary.

Poultice

A poultice or cataplasm is a preparation of herbs to be applied directly to the skin, or with a cloth. To make it, herbs are crushed, chopped, ground, pulverized, or turned into a paste for topical application. It might be heated. It is used to heal injuries on the skin. The disadvantage is that it takes longer for the desired effect compared to other topicals like oils, and it is messier to prepare.

Glycerite

Glycerite uses herb-infused glycerin to extract properties. The benefit of glycerin is that it can help hydrate the skin. While tinctures can be used, they might be irritating to the skin because of their acidity. Glycerite can be a great alternative for both its medical and beauty enhancement properties.

Carrier Oil

A carrier oil is an oil that can be applied topically and used for dilute extracts like essential oils. Essential oils can be very irritating to the skin. There is a wide range of carrier oils (Sweet Almond Oil; Jojoba Oil; Rosehip Oil; Fractionated Coconut Oil; Argan Oil; Grapeseed Oil; Avocado Oil; Neem Oil; Borage Oil and more), and the one used is determined by the ailment and the oil's properties. Carrier oil might be used as a way to treat a skin issue or to absorb essential oil into the skin.

Salve versus Balm versus Ointment

An ointment is a medical lotion. It is meant to be absorbed into the skin. Salve is a type of thick ointment that is usually infused with herbs. Balms are thick and sit on the skin as a barrier. Salves and balms usually are made of beeswax. Typically, they're fairly simple to make by adding beeswax, oil, and herbs.

Liniments and Emollients

Liniments are thin, water-like topicals, meant to be rubbed in as part of the treatment to relieve pain and stiffness. An emollient is a moisturizing treatment that is then covered to lock in the moisture.

Soap

Soap is used in unison with water for cleaning. There has been a recent surge in independent soap making. Soap is made typically from animal fat (tallow) or oil, lye and water. Making your own soap that is infused with herbs can be a good way to maintain long-term herbal skin treatment.

Compress versus Fomentation

A compress is a cloth applying pressure to the skin. It is dry or wet, hot or cold, and is used to relieve pain. A fomentation is a compress with a lotion, salve, poultice, etc. that is rubbed in.

Therapeutic Baths

Balneotherapy is the medical term for using bathing as a way to relieve ailments. It uses a combination of soaking and added herbs.

The method in which you choose to prepare your herbs is dependent on what you want to treat. You don't need to make a complicated elixir for everything. After a long day at work, if you're looking for a way to relax, a simple herbal tea might be everything you need. In the next chapter, we will look at how to make some of these concoctions.

Chapter Five

Creating Your Own Herbal Remedies Part Three: Recipes

This chapter is a collection of recipes. They are specific but flexible. This means that you can use the herbs suitable to you based on availability, preference, or instinct. These recipes outline the equipment, steps, dosage, and safety. If you are changing something in the recipe, make sure to be cautious and consider how herbs interact with each other.

As we amass this mountain of knowledge, we can now identify plants, build a raw ingredient inventory, and know some of the ways we can use them. In this chapter, we will look at some more in-depth practical uses of these remedies. Stepping away from theory, we need to consider the most effective ways of preparing these herbs. As a beginner, and even as a long-term herbalist, throwing a bunch of herbs into a pot is not effective, nor is it safe. This chapter is a collection of recipes that are proven safe and effective.

Before trying any recipe, make sure you are aware of how you may react to these plants. There could be plants you may not be aware you are allergic to or plants that interfere with your medications. Home remedies are for treating smaller ailments, but these are still medical ingredients. Many of these plants can cause harm if over-consumed. If you are pregnant, make sure to check with a doctor before using any alternative medicine.

Note: Use a thermometer if you desire. For reference,

low heat is 200–250 degrees F,

simmer is about 190–205 degrees F,

and boiling is 212 degrees F.

Remedies for Allergies

Garlic and Ginkgo Resin Syrup

This recipe reduces inflammation and allergy symptoms.

Ingredients

- 2 cups of water
- 2 ounces of chopped garlic
- 2 ounces of chopped ginkgo biloba
- ½ cup boney

How to prepare:

- Simmer the ingredients (except the honey) until half the pan has evaporated
- Take the herbage out and add the honey, simmer for 3 minutes
- Pour the solution into a jar and keep in the refrigerator

How to use:

Take 1 tablespoon 2–4 times a day during a flare-up to reduce allergy symptoms.

Allergy Topical

Ingredients

- 1 tsp chamomile
- 1 tsp peppermint
- 1 tsp comfrey
- 8 tbsp witch hazel
- 1–2 blackberries
- 1 cup 40% alcohol

How to prepare:

- Collect and chop fresh or dried herbs
- With a mortar and pestle, crush blackberries
- Add to the alcohol, and seal
- Infuse for 1 week
- Strain plant material
- Add to spray bottle

How to use:

- Spray the affected area lightly when needed 1–2 times a day

Allergy Symptoms Decoction

Ingredients

- 1 tsp mint

- 1–3 blackberries
- 1 tsp chamomile
- 2 cups water

How to prepare:

- Collect and chop fresh or dried herbs.
- In a mortar and pestle, crush blackberries
- Simmer in water for 15 minutes
- Let cool in the refrigerator for 1–2 hours

How to use:

- Serve with honey and ice to taste
- Feel the cooling mint soothe

Remedies for Respiratory Ailments

Mullein Decoction

Ingredients

- 2–3 tbsp mullein
- 1 tbsp elecampane
- 1 tbsp thyme
- 1/4 cup honey
- 5 cups water

How to Prepare:

- Since this is a tonic for respiratory health, embrace the steam during the cooking phase. This steam can help decongest mucus as well as moisten the airways.
- Put the herbs and honey in the water, and let simmer for 15–20 minutes as you enjoy the smell and feel of the steam. (Be careful steam is hot.)

- Serve hot or cold

How to use:

- Serve while hot and continue to inhale the steam as you go.

Mint Oil

This remedy can be made as an herb-infused oil, or the carrier oil might be used to dilute essential oils. Essential oils are more shelf-stable and have a much higher potency, but the problem is they are also very expensive. The alternative is infused oil, which may last only a few days, but gets the job done for cheaper. It takes a while for herbs to infuse, so if this is a remedy for flu season, you can make a batch a little beforehand to prepare.

Ingredients

- 1 tbsp peppermint leaves or 3-4 drops of essential oil
- (optional) 1-2 drops of eucalyptus oil
- ¼ cup carrier oil of choice

How to Prepare:

- For essential oils, just add a few drops to the carrier oil
- For infused oil, add herbs to the oil, and let infuse for a month

How to use:

- Apply to the chest, neck, and wrists.
- Inhale the aromatherapy, feel the cooling mint

Hot Compress/Bath

Ingredients

- Your choice of strong aromatic herbs (safe for topical use)
- Steamy Bath
- Mesh Bag (to hold herbs for easy clean up)
- A towel

How to Prepare:

- Draw a steamy bath and add aromatic herbs.
- Get a hot compress or water bottle (do not use a heating pad or anything electric in the bathtub)
- Get in the bath and place the towel on your chest, then the hot compress
- Inhale the steam and the smells
- Relax and let the compress and the bath soothe your respiratory discomfort

Horehound Electuary

Horehound is used for lung muscle spasms, coughing and mucus.

Ingredients

- 1:1 horehound to honey
- Lemon for taste

How to Prepare:

- Grind up dried horehound and mix it into your honey
- Take a tablespoon like you take cough syrup for relief

Remedies for Maintaining Wellness

St. John's Wort Herbal Tea to Fight Anxiety and Depression

Ingredients

- 1 cup of water
- 2 teaspoons St. John's wort
- 1 teaspoon honey (for taste)

How to Prepare:

- Simply boil the water and pour it into a mug that contains the herb
- Place plate over the mug to cover escaping steam
- Steep for 12 minutes
- Allow cooling before drinking

How to use:

- Find a place to relax, sip the tea
- Inhale the steam as you enjoy the drink

- Take once a day

Fragrant Oils for Clarity

<u>Ingredients</u>

- 1 tsp rosemary
- 1 tsp spruce needles
- 1 tsp pine needles
- 1 tsp bergamot
- ¼ cup favorite topical carrier oil

<u>How to Prepare:</u>

- Grind or chop herbs and add to a carrier oil in a sealable jar
- Store to infuse for 1 month
- Strain herbs
- Add to the rollable bottle

<u>How to use:</u>

- Roll oil on wrists, hands, neck, and chest
- Take deep breaths in to ground yourself for well-being

Liniment Oil

<u>Ingredients</u>

- 1 cup rose petals **OR** chamomile **OR** comfrey **OR** ginger **OR** St. John's wort **OR** yarrow
- 1 cup of favorite topical oil

<u>How to Prepare:</u>

- Add petals/leaves to the oil, seal the bottle and store
- Let infuse for 24 hours
- Strain plant material
- Store in refrigerator

How to use:

- Pour oil into hand to warm up
- Starting at your feet, slowly massage the oil into your body, really taking the time to feel each knot and sensation
- Take this time to check in with yourself, get to know what is going on with your body, and note a feeling of gratitude for your body and all that it does
- If you are putting oil on the bottom of your feet, make sure you put socks on after for safety
- You can also have someone else help you rub this oil into places like your back that you can't reach

---

Mental Grounding Tincture

Ingredients

- 1 tbsp sage
- ½ tsp dandelion
- ½ tsp parsley
- ¾ cups alcohol

How to Prepare:

- Grind fresh or dry herbs and add to alcohol
- Let infuse for 1–2 months, agitate regularly
- Strain and add to dropper bottle

How to use:

- Use this tincture as part of your mental wellness routine by taking 1-2 drops in the morning on the tongue or in a glass of water

Remedies for Digestive Problems

Overall Digestion Wellness Tincture

This remedy takes the form of a tincture so that it is fast-acting. This tincture is a build-it-yourself recipe that lets you pick the herbs you prefer or have access to. Whatever issues you are having, you might need heartburn relief, or want to steer away from anything that can act as a laxative.

Ingredients:

Alcohol

Digestive herbs like ginger, chamomile, fennel, and plantain 1:1:1:1

How to prepare:

- Add herbs to 40% alcohol and infuse for 1-2 months
- Add to dropper bottle

- Store up to 10 months
- Take 1–2 drops daily for overall digestive health

Digestion Kombucha

As we have learned in previous chapters on kombucha's ability to preserve herbs as part of its fermentation process, it is also a great choice for digestive treatments because of the probiotics, which aid in gut health. If you do not want to make kombucha, you may consider fermenting in honey alone. Shelf life is 1–3 months, once prepared and kept refrigerated.

Ingredients

- Scoby
- 6 black or green tea bags
- 1 cup sugar (not honey)
- 1 cup kombucha starter
- 14 cups water<u>redients</u>
- Scoby
- 6 black or green tea bags
- 1 cup sugar (not honey)
- 1 cup kombu
- Digestive herbs of choice

How to prepare:

- In a large pot, boil water
- Once boiling, add sugar until dissolved
- Add tea and herbs and steep for 10 minutes
- Allow to cool down completely before the next steps
- Add tea to jar with scoby

- Cover securely with cheesecloth and store in a cool, dark space for 6–11 days
- At this point, taste test, it should be slightly tart. Too tart and it has over fermented; not tart enough means it needs to ferment more.
- Strain kombucha and put it in a sealed container, to ferment 2 more days

How to use:

- You can serve your kombucha cold and even add some berries or lemon for health and taste
- You may be able to drink up to 2 cups daily

Laxative Tea

While the first steps in aiding constipation are drinking water, eating fiber, moving around, or drinking coffee, you might want extra aid in finding relief. You can make alterations to this recipe as you see fit, to make the tea to your liking.

1 teaspoon of leaves to 6 ounces of water is the tea standard. Whether you make this a dry mixture or add them as separate ingredients is up to you. Adding them separately might allow for alterations of the recipe as you see fit. You may start 1:1:1:1 and discover what you need to alter for your body.

Ingredients

- Dried dandelion root
- Chamomile
- Roasted chicory root

How to prepare:

- Chicory roots must be made into a decoction by adding it to water, bringing it to a boil, and simmering for 5 minutes
- Take off the heat and add the other herbs
- Steep for 5–10 minutes
- Strain, or remove the tea infuser
- Add honey to taste

Diarrhea Treatment

Diarrhea is not only unpleasant, but it can be very dangerous when left untreated. The first major point is to make sure that you stay hydrated, as diarrhea causes a high loss of liquids. If you keep on top of overall health, you may prevent these episodes, but this recipe is to help when maintenance is overruled by other factors.

This recipe could be made as tea or a prepared tincture. When treating diarrhea as a symptom, you are not necessarily treating the overall cause, and it might be a good sign your body is reacting. These cures soothe your stomach and try to stop your body from reacting so drastically and causing other problems.

Ingredients

- Lemon balm and chamomile
- Thyme **OR** Oregon grape **OR** raspberry/blackberry leaves.
- Ginger

How to prepare:

- If you are making this remedy on the spot for fast relief, bring water to a boil, remove it from heat
- Add 1 tsp of leaves to 6 ounces of water and steep for 10 minutes, remove infuser to strain

- Add lemon for taste as well as its antibacterial, antiviral properties

OR

- Add an even ratio of each ingredient to 40% alcohol or stronger
- Let infuse for 1–2 months, store for up to 10 months
- Take a few drops when necessary

Remedies for Stress and Anxiety

Lavender and Chamomile Oil to Relax

Ingredients

- 2 tbsp lavender, herbs or essential oil
- 2 tbsp chamomile, herbs or essential oil
- ½ cup of favorite topical carrier oil

How to Prepare:

- If you are using essential oils, simply add a few drops to your carrier oil
- If you are infusing an oil, add your herbs to your oil of choice
- Seal and infuse for 1–2 months, shaking regularly
- Strain plant matter
- You might want to dilute this infused oil more
- Add to roller

How to use:

- Keep on your bedside table
- Roll onto wrists, or palms of hands at night
- Bring it close enough to your face to smell. Close your eyes, take deep breaths, and relax

---

Thyme and Chamomile Oxymel For Stress and Anxiety

Ingredients

- 2 tbsp thyme
- 2 tbsp chamomile
- Honey
- Apple cider vinegar

How to Prepare:

- The amount of honey to vinegar is your choice, ranging from 1:1 to 5:1, depending on your preference. It should equal ¾ cup in total
- Add honey, herbs, and vinegar to a jar. Seal and shake 1-2 times a week for 2 weeks
- Strain plant material
- Store 6 months

How to use:

- Take 1-2 tbsp straight or add to a calming tea
- Take a minute or two to smell the calming scent
- Take a few deep breaths

Skullcap and Mugwort Herbal Cigarette for Nerves

Smoking is not for everyone, nor is it encouraged. This is a good alternative for those who are trying to smoke less, want an alternative to regular cigarettes or want a smokable option for reducing anxiety.

Ingredients

- 2 tbsp mullein
- ½ tbsp mugwort
- ½ tbsp skullcap
- ½ tbsp lavender or mint for taste
- Rolling paper
- Filter

How to Prepare:

- Grind up the herbs
- Take a rolling paper of your choice and filter, or add it to a pipe

How to use:

- Find a place you are comfortable and allowed to smoke
- Use as a calming alternative to tobacco cigarettes
- Not intended for chain-smoking

Lemon Balm and Valerian Tea for Sleep

Valerian is not meant for long-time use.

Ingredients

- ½ tbsp valerian Root
- ½ tbsp lemon balm
- 1 cup water

How to Prepare:

- Boil water, take off the heat and pour over herbs
- Steep 1–2 minutes

How to use:

- Serve as desired, with lemon or honey

Remedies for Beauty Care

Everyday Beauty Toner

Distilled rose water is used as a toner and can even be drunk (for its antioxidants). It can soothe skin and the antioxidants are beneficial as an astringent for everyday maintenance. Distilling is typically better than steeping as it is pure and sterilized, which is better when putting on the skin. Lasts 6 months in the refrigerator.

Ingredients

- Rose petals and water 1:1 (4 cups loose roses to 4 cups water makes about 2 cups yield)
- (Other skin beneficial herbs of choice, such as lavender, chamomile, etc.)
- Note: All types of roses can work in this recipe, but some roses are preferred. Wild rose bush varieties popular in New England are a good choice.

How to prepare:

- Start by removing all excess material from the flower petals
- Thoroughly rinse the rose petals under cold water
- Use sterilized dishes for best results
- Place rose petals in water in a distillation pot (use a large pot, with a brick or platform to lift a heat safe container inside.)
- Turn heat on to the lowest temperature that creates steam
- Put the domed lid on the pot upside down. This will cause the condensation to pool at the bottom and into the heat safe container to catch. Make sure that the condensation drip and the container align properly.
- Use ice cubes to occasionally cool the lid to encourage condensation.
- This might take a while (about 30 minutes), but you should not boil until all the water in the petals is gone.
- Let cool
- Remove the catching container, and put rosewater in a sterilized, sealable container
- You might filter the plant material out of any remaining water and use it if desired as a rose decoction

How to use:

- Use 1-2 times daily during skin care routine
- With a cotton ball or similar, dampen slightly and lightly apply to the skin

Rosemary/Nettle Hair Oil

Ingredients

- 2 tbsp rosemary **OR** nettle
- ¼ cup argan Oil

How to Prepare:

- Grind rosemary and add to oil
- Seal and let infuse for 1 month, agitate regularly
- Strain plant matter and store

How to use:

- Add a few drops of oil to a spray bottle
- Dilute with water
- Spray onto the roots of the hair 4 times a week

Herbal Soap for Skin Wellness

Some people may be able to make soap from scratch, but this recipe uses a pure version of soap as a base.

Ingredients

- 1 tbsp lavender
- 1 tbsp yarrow
- 1 tbsp cornflower
- 1 tbsp glycerin
- 1 cup oil of choice (olive oil, jojoba, or sunflower oil is recommended)

- 1 tsp ground oatmeal
- 1 tbsp honey
- 1 lb soap base

How to Prepare:

- Melt premade soap blocks into a slow cooker and wait until melted
- Add your desired oils, herbs, exfoliants, and fragrances
- Essential oils don't take well to heat, so add them in, stir, and start pouring into molds
- Herbs might not have enough time to infuse into the soap, so to ensure the benefits are optimal, you may infuse your carrier oil with these herbs instead, and only add the herbs as a visual or exfoliant appeal
- Pour the soap into molds and use for hands or body wash

Herbal Baths for Skin and Hair

Ingredients

- 2 tbsp rosemary
- 2 tbsp stinging nettle
- 2 tbsp burdock root

How to Prepare:

- Draw a bath to your liking
- In the kitchen, boil water and make a concentration for your bath; this helps reduce mess and ensures that everything has been extracted
- Add concentrate and any other materials to the bath

- If adding any oils, remember that this can cause the bath to be very slippery and dangerous. When you are done, ensure you rinse out the tub before the next person
- In the bath, use a cloth or loofah to exfoliate

Facial Poultice for Healthy Skin

<u>Ingredients</u>

- ½ cup aloe
- 2 tbsp rose petals
- ½ tbsp yarrow
- ½ tbsp chickweed

<u>How to Prepare:</u>

- In a blender or with a mortar and pestle, grind the herbs into fairly fine sizes. This will help ensure even concentration, and it will stay on easier as the mask works
- Combine the mix of herbs with some liquid that is water-based, like rose water. It is best not to use alcohol, thick oils, or too much glycerin on your face
- The mixture should be the consistency of a thinner paste

<u>How to use:</u>

- Apply a thin layer to your face
- Let sit for 10 minutes, then wash off
- Repeat every 2 weeks

Remedies for Inflammation

Green Tea and Oxymel Tonic for Inflammation

Ingredients

- 1 bag of green tea
- ½ tsp white willow bark
- ½ tbsp black pepper
- Honey
- Apple cider vinegar

How to Prepare:

- The amount of honey to vinegar is your choice, ranging from 1:1 to 5:1, depending on your preference. It should equal ¾ cup in total
- Add honey, herbs, and vinegar to a jar. Seal and shake 1–2 times a week for 2 weeks
- Strain plant material

- Store 6 months

How to use:

- Take 1 tbsp for inflammation as needed directly or dilute in water

---

Meadowsweet Liniment for Topical Inflammation

Ingredients

- 1 cup witch hazel
- 4 tbsp meadowsweet
- 2 tbsp yarrow
- 2 tbsp comfrey
- 1 tbsp carrier oil

How to Prepare:

- Grind herbs together, add to the jar
- Pour alcohol over top and seal
- Infuse for 1 month, shake 2–3 times a week
- Strain plant material
- Store in bottle and add oil

How to use:

- Shake the bottle to mix alcohol and oil
- In your hand pour a tablespoon of liquid
- On an inflamed area, use this liquid to massage the area
- Liniments absorb quickly, but the massage can help the blood flow to the area
- Repeat as needed

Remedies for Minor Wounds and Bruises

Pine Resin Salve

This salve is for reducing inflammation and pain. Pine sap is antibacterial and can fight infections. Also, it can draw out slivers. Pine resin is very flammable, so be cautious when using it. Pine sap can be very hard to work with, so use oil or alcohol to get it off of equipment. You may want to set aside equipment just to deal with sap. Soft sap might be quicker to dissolve in oil, but dry sap can be crushed into a powder, which makes removing impurities easier. The shelf life is 6–9 months.

Note: Before starting this recipe, take note that dissolving resin into oil can take up to 12 hours to render.

Pine sap, resin, and pitch: Sap is like liquid honey, and it's for the regular circulation of the tree. Pitch is like crystalized honey; it is a defense mechanism for the tree when there is damage. Resin is solid and hard pitch.

Ingredients

- ¼ cup white pine resin
- ½ cup oil (use preferred topical oil, olive oil works fine)
- ½ ounce beeswax (add more for thicker consistency)
- Use other herbs as desired

Equipment needed

- Double boiler (A pot inside a pot with water in between. This means the heat is evenly distributed, and not directly on the ingredients.)

How to prepare:

- Prepare the pine resin/pitch. If you are able to crush hard resin into a powder, do so. Removing impurities when in liquid form is difficult. If there are impurities at the end of the pine/oil infusion, you can strain through a cheesecloth.
- You may use a slow cooker for this process for double boiling the pine and oil so that it can be heated longer. Add water to the middle section between pots.
- Turn on to gentle heat
- Occasionally check on the mixture, and give it a stir when needed. 1–12 hours
- If there are impurities, strain and put back into the pot
- Add beeswax, melt
- Pour into a sterile, sealable container and label

How to use:

- Use as a topical lotion on all minor external injuries such as cuts and bruises.
- Absorbs quickly. A little goes a long way.

Healing Ice Fomentation for Bruising

Ingredients

- 1/2 tbsp yarrow
- ¼ tbsp chamomile
- ½ white willow bark
- 1 cup water
- 1 towel

How to Prepare:

- In a pot, heat the water and herbs to create a decoction for 10 minutes
- Take off the heat and let cool

How to use:

- Dip a towel in the cool liquid and apply to area
- Cool temperature helps with swelling. If needed, throw the towel inside the freezer for a few minutes

Lavender Tincture for Wounds

Ingredients

- 2 tbsp lavender
- ¼ cup 40% alcohol

How to Prepare:

- Add the herbs to the alcohol, seal, and let infuse for 2 weeks
- Shake every 1–2 days
- Strain plant matter from liquid
- Add to dropper bottle

How to use:

- Add a drop or two to minor wounds to prevent infection 1–2 times a day

Remedies for Regulating Blood Pressure

Pepper and Turmeric Shot

Ingredients

- 1 tsp turmeric
- ½ tsp fresh ground pepper
- 1 tbsp lemon juice or apple cider vinegar
- 1 tbsp water

How to Prepare:

- Add all of the ingredients together and take a shot, or add to other drinks.
- Take once daily for healthy blood pressure management.

Potassium Tea for High Blood Pressure (with honey)

Ingredients

- 1 tbsp, 1:1:1:1 dandelion, nettle, mint, lotus root
- 1 cup water

How to Prepare:

- Bring water to a boil, pour over herbs
- Serve as desired, with honey

Periwinkle Root Tincture for Low Blood Pressure

Ingredients

- 1 tbsp Periwinkle root
- 1 cup water

How to Prepare:

- Boil water and root for 10 minutes

How to use:

- Drink to help low blood pressure days. **Do not drink every day, it may cause miscarriage.**
- Add cinnamon and honey to taste

Remedies for Treating Infections

Anti-Microbial Tea

Ingredients

- 1 tbsp ginger
- 1 lemon slice
- 1 cup water

How to Prepare:

- Boil water, pour over ginger
- Squeeze in lemon, drink 2 times a day

Electuary For Infection

Ingredients

- 1 tbsp of 1:1:1:2, ginger, thyme, sage, basil, fresh garlic,
- 1 tbsp honey

How to Prepare:

- Grind or crush herbs and add to honey

How to use:

- Take a spoonful by mouth when fighting internal infection
- Serve alone for mouth and throat infections, or as an additive to tea

---

Honey Poultice for Skin Infection

Ingredients

- 1 tbsp honey

How to Prepare:

- Add pure honey to the site of an injury to fight infection, bacteria, and fungus, and promote healing

How to use:

- Use 1-2 times daily as you change bandages and clean the site

---

Salve for Drawing out Infection

Ingredients

- 1 tbsp activated charcoal

- 5 tbsp infused oil of lavender, comfrey, plantain, and calendula
- 1 tbsp beeswax (adjust for thickness)
- 2 tbsp bentonite or kaolin clay

How to Prepare:

- Infuse oil in a double boiler for an hour or naturally for 1–2 weeks
- Strain herbs
- Melt beeswax in a pot, add oil
- Take off heat, add charcoal and clay
- Stir until dry for a smooth consistency
- Add to sterilized jar, label

How to use:

- Clean site of infection well
- Add a layer of salve before bed to draw out the infection
- Clean off in the morning, bandage or let breathe
- Repeat if necessary
- Store up to 2 years

Oils for Treating Wounds

Ingredients

- ¼ cup coconut oil (antibacterial)
- 3 tbsp lavender, sage, thyme, rosemary 1:1:1:1

How to Prepare:

- Melt coconut oil in a pot at low temperature and add herbs
- Let infuse for an hour, and strain

- Remove from heat, and stir the oil. Coconut oil is solid at room temperature, so it can't infuse as well naturally. Stirring as it cools will allow oil to be a creamy texture and be easier to use.
- Add to jar and keep in refrigerator or freezer

How to use:

- If you have a topical skin infection with unbroken skin, add some of this oil morning and night to fight bacteria and encourage healing

Garlic Tincture

Ingredients

- 1:2 garlic to alcohol

How to Prepare:

- Chop or crush garlic and add it to the alcohol
- Leave for 1 month to infuse
- Strain, leave for another day or two
- Add to dropper bottle

How to use:

- Garlic tincture can be used as a way to fight topical infections and promote healing by adding 1-2 drops to the area 1-2 times a day
- Internally, garlic tincture can be consumed for infections, up to 5 drops a day

Remedies for Bloating

Dandelion Tea for Bloating

<u>Ingredients</u>

- 2 tsp dried dandelion (root, leaf, or flower)
- 1 cup water

<u>How to Prepare:</u>

- Boil water
- Take off the heat and add tea leaves
- Let steep for 5–10 minutes

<u>How to use:</u>

- Serve as desired when bloated

Fennel and Chamomile Tincture

Ingredients

- ½ cup 40% alcohol
- 1 tbsp fennel
- 1 tbsp chamomile

How to Prepare:

- Grind or chop herbs and combine with alcohol
- Let infuse for 6–10 weeks
- Strain plant materials
- Add to dropper bottle

How to use:

- Take 3–4 drops straight or diluted in water whenever you feel bloated

Lemon Balm Oxymel

Ingredients

- Honey
- Raw apple cider vinegar
- ¼ cup dried lemon balm

How to Prepare:

- The amount of honey to vinegar is your choice, ranging from 1:1 to 5:1, depending on your preference, it should equal ¾ cup in total

- Add honey, herbs, and vinegar to a jar. Seal and shake 1–2 times a week for 2 weeks.
- Strain plant material
- Store 6 months

How to use:

- Take a tablespoon directly, or add it to your drink of choice when looking to reduce bloating

Remedies for Insect Bites, Stings, and Rashes

Plantain Poultice (Quick Relief)

Ingredients

- 1 tbsp plantain
- 1–2 tbsp water
- optional ½–1 tbsp clay and/or charcoal

How to Prepare:

- If you are outside with no other option, chew a plantain leaf to create a paste and apply to the skin
- If you are able, crushing the plantain leaf, adding clean water, and the optional clay or charcoal to create the paste is more hygienic

Yarrow Healing Salve

Ingredients

- Optional: calendula, lavender, lemon balm
- 1½ cups fresh yarrow leaves (anti-inflammatory, anti-itch, antibacterial, stops bleeding)
- 2 tbsp beeswax
- Topical oil of your choice (like jojoba or olive)

How to Prepare:

- In a bottle, mix your oil and herbs (make sure the oil completely covers the herbs). Seal and let infuse for a month OR mix oil and herbs in a double boiler, and leave on gentle heat overnight.
- Strain out plant debris
- In a double boiler, add the 1 cup of infused oil and beeswax until melted
- Pour into a sterilized, sealable container and label (shelf-stable 1 year)

How to use:

- Apply a thin layer to the area when needed
- In a pinch, use a poultice of yarrow to relieve irritation or bleeding, and use salve as follow-up treatment

Oatmeal Relief Bath

Oatmeal baths are soothing to irritated skin and also reduce itching.

Ingredients

- ½–1 ½ cups oatmeal
- Up to 8 tbsp of herbs: thyme, mint, rose, rosemary

How to Prepare:

- Run a bath to your liking. In the kitchen, put the oatmeal in a blender and blend it into flour.
- In a pot of 4–6 cups of water, bring to boil, and set aside 1 cup of hot water
- Add oatmeal, to create a sort of concentrated oat milk, and strain
- In the cup of hot water, you can add herbs to make a concentrated tea. These steps reduce the amount of debris in the bathtub for cleaning.
- Pour these concentrates into the bath
- Relax, soak for 30 minutes

Mint Aloe Soothing Lotion

Ingredients

- 2 tbsp aloe
- 2 tbsp mint
- ¼ cup water
- ¼ tbsp beeswax
- 2 ▫ tbsp carrier oil (recommended sunflower or jojoba)
- (Optional: add rosemary in with mint for bug bite relief.)

How to Prepare:

- In a pinch, you can combine aloe (store-bought or harvested) and the mint in a blender and apply, especially to kids who need relief quicker
- 1-2 days before making add the mint to the oil to encourage extraction
- In a pot, melt beeswax at low temperature; when melted, add infused oil, water, and aloe slowly (so as not to harden wax)
- Keep stirring on low heat until fully incorporated
- Remove from heat, stir frequently as lotion cools to keep light
- Store in refrigerator

How to use:

- Before you spend time outside or in the sun, if you know you are going to be around anything irritating to your skin, it is a good idea to stock up on this recipe
- Whenever there is skin irritation, add this lotion as an instant reliever
- Reapply as needed

Moisturizing Glycerite for Healing

Glycerin is used as a hydrator. This can be important in the healing process of all skin damage. As the healing process creates new skin, the damaged skin dries, causing pain and itching.

Ingredients

- 2 tsp comfrey petals
- 2 tsp marshmallow petals or root
- 2 tsp rose petals

- 2 tsp echinacea petal or roots or Turmeric Ground
- ½ cup glycerin

How to Prepare:

- Combine herbs and glycerin in a sterilized, sealable container
- Infuse for 3–7 weeks, shaking every day or so
- Strain plant pieces
- Shelf-stable up to 5 years

How to use:

- Use a thin layer of infused glycerin over the area of dry skin
- If you are using another topical along with this process, such as a salve, wait until the glycerin has soaked in, then seal with a hydrophobic salve
- Repeat once daily until healed
- It is not recommended to overuse glycerin, as over-hydrating the skin can do damage to the healing process

Other Remedies

Earaches:

Blue vervain tea, steeped for 10 minutes

Energy/Strength

Ingredients

- ½ cup 40% alcohol
- 2 tbsp feverfew

How to Prepare:

- Grind or chop herbs and combine with alcohol
- Let infuse for 6–10 weeks
- Strain plant materials
- Add to dropper bottle

How to use:

- Take 3-4 drops straight or diluted in water midday to help midday fatigue

---

Mouthwash

Ingredients

- ½ cup 40% alcohol
- 2 tbsp peppermint

How to Prepare:

- Grind or chop herbs and combine with alcohol
- Let infuse for 6-10 weeks
- Strain plant materials

Headache

Ingredients

- 2 tbsp willow bark
- 1 tsp catnip
- 1 tsp skullcap
- 1 cup water

How to Prepare:

- Boil willow bark in water for 10 minutes
- Take off the heat and add the rest of the herbs

How to use:

- Make a cup of tea whenever you have a headache
- Drink in a quiet dark room

Menstrual Issues Tea

Ingredients

- 2 tbsp primrose
- 1 tsp raspberry
- 1 cup water

How to Prepare:

- Boil water
- Take off the heat and add the herbs
- Steep for 10 minutes

How to use:

- Make a cup of tea whenever necessary for cramps and other symptoms

UTI (Urinary Tract Infection) Tincture

Ingredients

- ½ cup 40% alcohol
- 1 tbsp stinging nettle
- 1 tbsp barberry

How to Prepare:

- Grind or chop herbs and combine with alcohol
- Let infuse for 2 weeks
- Strain plant materials
- Add to dropper bottle

How to use:

- Take 10 drops daily until you're healed

There is an ever-expanding collection of useful remedies. Using herbal remedies in companionship with pharmaceutical treatments is the best way to keep you and your family healthy. As you add more information to your inventory of knowledge, you will become a master without realizing it. The best part about these recipes is that they are already in your cupboard or backyard. Feel free to use your knowledge of plants to alter these recipes for what works or is available to you.

Chapter Six

Foraging for Medicinal Herbs in New England

This chapter is a beginner's guide to safe and proper forging and gathering of your medicinal plants. Forging is the cheapest and quickest way to build an inventory—especially if you know what you are looking for.

There are lots of benefits to getting a plant from out in nature, even if it is simply being outdoors getting exercise. But there are a lot of things to know before you start consuming foraged plants. Therefore, this chapter comes after the ones on preparing herbs. It is better to prepare and get used to store-bought herbs, then slowly move into foraging and gathering what you are comfortable with later in your practice.

The act of foraging puts into action all the information that you know about the plants from theory. When we think about what we know about plants, it can take a while to put it into practice. Nature is unpredictable and the conditions in which you find plants are going to be different every time. Reference photos are absolutely necessary when you find a plant and need to know what it is and if it is usable. But how do you know where to look?

Foraging might not look the way you picture. We can romanticize what we are going to do before we do it, but in action, it doesn't work. Foraging might sound like an adventure in the woods that marvelously turns into a foraging event. What a beginner needs to know, in the city or in the country, is that you learn where things grow and go to it. You don't just haphazardly find rosemary growing on the first path you choose. If you know where and when to look and go out with the intention of foraging, you might find a lot more success.

Sometimes foraging does just spontaneously happen. As you learn to identify plants, and better yet, learn to identify the plants that you need, you are going to be aware all the time of the plants around you. This is important because one day when you are out walking your dog you might notice a white birch, ripe with catkins. You might not always be prepared at the moment, but take notes of where these desirable plants are for future foraging. In my experience of foraging, I look for the tall, dill-looking, overgrown asparagus bushes in the late summer months. By the time it looks like this, it is way past eating, but it is a lot easier to notice than the small stalks in the spring. By then, I will return to where I last saw them.

Advantages of Foraging

- Being outside
- Organic
- Trust sourcing and quality
- You can save money

How to Forage in your Area

On your first few rounds of foraging, you may or may not be able to find the plants you want or need. Observing your local area, though, is a great way to build a foundation. You might be foraging locally, as in your neighborhood. This might mean you get familiar with the kinds of plants that are growing in the ditches and what kinds of conditions are around. If you are relocating to certain areas for their desirable conditions, you might take some time to get familiar with the area as well.

Even if you have permission to forage, or the land you are foraging on is open to the public, always do your research, and triple-check with your local government and conservation authorities about what pesticides, herbicides, or other chemicals have been used. Even if it has been a few years since being sprayed, these chemicals can last a long time in the ground. If you are in ditches, or even close to farmland, be conscious of the possibility that there are things on those plants that you do not know of. Even if you are absolutely sure, make sure to soak your harvest in a mixture of water and apple cider vinegar for as long as possible to make sure you are as safe as you can be.

15 Tips on how to Safely Forage for Medicinal Herbs

1. Being able to identify your target herb/plant accurately is crucial. Get an idea of what your plant looks like in the wild, as well as where it might grow (near specific trees, near water, etc.).
2. Some plants look similar but are very different from each other. Research your plant before you go out, and what it looks like in your area. How can you tell the difference between it and something else, and is the similar plant dangerous?

3. Know what part of the plant you need, to reduce waste and encourage regrowth. You most likely don't need the whole plant or all of the plants. Take what you need and be kind.

4. Some plants are only edible in moderation. While weeds can be plentiful and it can be great to pick more to allow competition from other plants, there are dangers to over-consuming plants.

5. Some plants are illegal to pick. Make sure the plants you are interested in are not endangered.

6. Let someone know what area you will be in, and if possible, the route you are going to take. Don't underestimate how easy it is to get lost.

7. Be conscious of animal competition. They live in the forest and don't have a grocery store alternative. Always leave some plants to repopulate, but if you notice something has been eating them, be kind. This keeps the environment supported for years of foraging to come.

8. Be aware of local laws against foraging.

9. Be aware of private property laws.

10. Have a plan and bring the right tools to support your foraging needs. Some plants are simple to pluck from the ground, but in many cases, it can be really difficult to break even small branches or dig up roots. It can protect you and also be less traumatic to a plant if you are only cutting pieces off with a knife instead of shredding it off with your hands.

11. Wash everything thoroughly. Even though you want to be working in a place without chemicals, you never know what has touched a plant. It can be fun to pick and eat, but it can be dangerous too.

12. Pick plants that look fresh and untouched. Not only is this important in the context of quality and potency, it is also important for your safety.

13. What reactions do you have to plants? It might be fun to rush into herbalism, but slowly adding plants and remedies into your life can help you determine whether you are reacting positively to these new plants.

14. Not everything can be eaten raw and not everything is used internally. As medicinal ingredients, you need to prepare everything as directed to prevent issues.

15. Use your intuition. Learn how to trust your gut. Always follow safety procedures, but also listen to your instincts. If you don't feel comfortable, don't do it.

Foraging gear

- Scissors or shears
- Canvas bag and Gloves
- Notebook, pen/pencil, or notes on your phone
- Camera (plant identifier app)
- This book

Have a list of what you are looking for. Be really specific if you are just starting and learning identification. Limiting yourself to three to four herbs at a time can reduce anxiety, mistakes, and can help build a deeper knowledge of these plants, one at a time. Be alert, focused, and observant. While it may be on the list, I want to reiterate the importance of gloves. I have had my fair share of stubbornness in not wearing gloves, but it really does not prove anything. Gloves are important for a lot of reasons, and physical and chemical dangers such as thorns and poison ivy are just a start. If you are spending a long day in the field, you don't want to get your hands dirty and be unable to wash them for hours on end. You might wade through the brush for certain herbs, and you don't know if there are sharp branches, bugs, snakes, or other animals in there that see your hand first.

When preparing to find these herbs, you might want to do research beforehand. Knowing how tall they are, what they look like this time of year, what they might look like in your area especially, whether they grow in small clusters, in bushes, out in the open, in the ditches, near rotting logs, acidic soil, etc., will help you find them. The weather and surroundings can make it appear a lot different from the photo. Depending on whether it is very sunny, overcast, out in the open, or under a tree will change the appearance of color dramatically.

Walk slowly. You are looking for herbs, and you might miss them if you are worried about getting your workout, too. Take pictures and notes of unfamiliar herbs so you can learn about them later; remember where you found the plants or note observations you want to remember for next time. There is so much to learn, and when you write things down, you are able to ensure that you create a long-term record of what you have used and harvested.

DOs

- Get permission to forage
- Let someone know you are out foraging
- Wear protective gear, this might include reflective gear, but also the right shoes and socks, thick pants (for thorns, brush), weather-appropriate clothing, protective gloves, bug and sun protection, etc.
- Learn to correctly identify plants and their similar counterparts

DON'Ts

- Harvest too much
- Harvest endangered or protected plants
- Take diseased, contaminated, or damaged plants

Plant Conservation

In the next chapter on gardening, we will look at what it means to have a garden, and the impact it has on the local environment. What species are introduced into the area has a huge effect on how successful native species are. The conservation of plant species is also a responsibility of the forager. As someone interested in foraging, you are probably also interested in making sure that this remains possible for years to come. New England as a whole is home to plants that are both globally and regionally rare. There are many things at play in the decrease in plant populations, including environmental issues and the loss of land, but some things remain in the hands of foragers.

The first rule in making sure that the plant populations thrive is first to be respectful of the environment around you. It is a legal requirement to make sure your personal litter is put in its proper waste container, but if you are able to carry the supplies for safe pickup, removing litter when you can from these places helps the entire ecosystem. If you are foraging on trials, try to leave everything the same as you found it, and leave the trail as little as possible. When you are actively foraging, try to be respectful of both other foragers and plant populations and take only what you need. Try to leave enough behind so that it can regrow or reseed. Be aware of endangered or rare plants, and the laws regarding what can and can't be harvested.

Chapter Seven

Cultivating Medicinal Plants at Home

The term field guide gives the impression of mysterious adventures of foraging in the wild, but this guide can also be of assistance when it comes to questions, concerns, and clarifications for those who want to bring medicinal plants closer to home. Growing herbs at home has advantages over purchasing and foraging. These advantages are having a sense of control over what you are growing, how much you are growing, and what happens to those plants. These can be hugely important factors for those who rely on the plants, as well as those who do not have access to information about whether an area of foraging space is purely organic. All three options (bought, foraged, garden-grown) have positives and negatives to them and do not need to be practiced separately.

Gardening, like foraging, has benefits that go beyond its product attributes. One of the greatest pleasures, according to countless testimonies, is gardening. Gardening or growing plants, in general, can create pride in watching something grow that you have taken care of, as well as being useful in cultivating usable ingredients.

There is also a huge amount of flexibility in the size and variation of growing plants that makes it accessible to almost everyone. When put together, herbalism and gardening are the perfect combinations. People are drawn to them individually because they provide agency and control over what people are putting in their bodies, for health benefits and monetary purposes. So, combining gardening and herbal healing not only makes sense to cultivate ingredients for herbalism but also because the disciplines share underlying objectives. In addition to growing supplies for herbal remedies, those who are also growing food are supporting their healing with fresh, unprocessed food that is denser in beneficial nutrients.

If you are someone who does not have obvious/explicit access to a personal garden, this does not exclude you from the conversation. One option is a community or allotment garden. A community garden is usually run as a group effort, making choices as a team. Community gardens are a great option for those who are open to socializing, who want to learn from other gardeners, and who appreciate or need help to take care of their garden. An allotment garden is a garden for rent that is for independent personal use. Allotment gardens might be a single garden or a collection of independent gardeners. These are great for people who want more control over their garden and prefer more solitude (at least for gardening). If these options are not available to you, talk to your local community center, private landowners/landlords, or to social media groups to see if starting one is an option. Gardens can also be grown in pots, on balconies, or even on windowsills.

Whenever you choose to plant something, it is important to question its interaction with the rest of the environment. The list of plants you might be able to forage in your area contains many invasive species, and many plants not originally native to the area. Just because you can find them in the area does not mean that you should try to plant them in your garden—chances are some of them will pop up there anyway. Double-check if a plant is going to be an issue for your garden or the community before planting. Even plants that are common in gardens for ornament, like yarrow, can be invasive. It might be as simple as making sure these plants don't spread and take or removing flowers before they turn to seedpods, or avoiding the plant altogether. Many invasive plants can damage the soil and suffocate the other, less competitive plants in your garden.

How to Plan a Home Garden as an Herbalist

We have talked previously about being a beginner in terms of herbalism, and how stressful it can be when it feels like there is so much to learn, and you don't know where to start. If you are someone who doesn't know much about plants besides sun and water, then the idea of growing these plants on top of that might seem like too much to bear. We also talked about how much easier it is to start identifying plants when you are able to focus/narrow down to your local plants, such as those that grow in New England. Growing can be simplified in the same way. You don't need to learn how to grow every plant, nor do you need to learn vague facts about gardening around the world. You are interested in herbalism and healing in New England, and this can give you a really solid start in being able to plan and make decisions.

Depending on what time of year you are reading this, you might feel more or less rushed to get going and grow. This rush can make us blind to informed decisions. You might just be getting started on both herbalism and gardening, on a time crunch to get plants in the ground in the spring and choose plants based on recognizing their names like basil or thyme. Nothing bad will happen, of course, but it might be irrelevant to your cause, and if you are using herbalism/gardening to save money, rushing in without a plan can be counterproductive. To narrow down what you want to grow, here are some things you need to consider:

- Do you plan on using a combination of foraging/buying? This choice is going to cross off herbs that you plan on sourcing outside of your garden.
- Is the point of your garden to be the main/only source of herbs? This will send you straight to your planned recipes to see what plants you need.
- There could be hundreds of herbs to grow at home, so decide on the ones most useful to you and your practice. Being realistic, what recipes are you going to try this year, and what do they need?
- If you have plants in mind: Is it the right time to plant them? (Some plants are planted in the fall.) How long does it take them to grow? Are they perennials or annuals? Do they complement the living situation you are in? (Size, soil type, moveable?)
- What will work with the space you have? Sometimes it isn't a question of what you want to do, but what you can do. How much is possible with the space you have?
- How much can you commit to? Gardening can be as little or as much as you intend. What is obtainable to you and your life?
- Niche and other goals. Are you passionate about native plants? You might not be interested in foraging, but still want to only grow plants that naturally grow locally.
- Invasive species. Just because something isn't native to an area, does not mean it is invasive, but it is still something to be conscious about.

Sourcing plants can be done locally or online. If you are interested in planting a native/local plant garden, you might be able to source transplanted plants, or even forage seeds.

Starting your Garden, Inside and Out

At this point, you might have an idea of what plants you want to grow, and where you will be growing them. But how to start and continue to care for your garden throughout the entire season? There are not a lot of steps to gardening, but the steps that exist can make it or break it. To prepare your garden, you will want to start with containers, soil, watering, and sun.

Pots

Get the right containers for your plants. A lot of the tips about growing herbs inside are standard for growing all indoor plants, but pots are different when it comes to herbs. There are a few reasons to plant herbs in pots, even outside. Some herbs, like mint, can be invasive, so keeping them in one place can reduce their spread. The other reason is some herbs do better in smaller spaces. Herbs can have shorter lifespans, which means you don't have as much time to perfect your care. For example, some plants prefer to be root-bound, and if the pot is too big it will spend its energy filling out the pot instead of growing foliage. If you are growing a spider plant that can be passed down from generation to generation, you have time to slowly build the plant up. Herbs need a pot that will allow them to grow bigger, but not overwhelm the plant. Up to eighteen inches deep to grow is a safe bet.

If you are getting a tree, or something taller you intend to keep in a pot, getting something sturdy (even something with wheels) is necessary. If you are growing plants inside with very limited space, make sure your pots fit on windowsills, or even hanging baskets near windows to ensure sunlight, or invest in a vertical garden. If you are planting outside, you might have a balance of things in pots and things directly in the ground. If you have space to keep your herbs outside in the summer, it can reduce the mess in the house as well as give them sunlight that you don't need to monitor.

It's important to find a balance between function and fashion when it comes to planting pots, especially if you are keeping them inside. Pick something that is going to last and look good in your home. Ceramic and terracotta are the preferred materials, as plastic can leach chemicals and it is typically not long-lasting. For almost every plant you have, making sure there is enough drainage is essential to making sure your plant survives. If you are inside, these drainage holes usually need a plate of some sort that catches excess water. This plate may or may not come with your pot.

Soil

If you are using a pot, most plants need well-draining soil as well as a well-drained pot. This, along with accurate pot size, reduces the chances of root rot. The best way to go is to get potting soil that is sterilized, meaning it does not carry diseases and is balanced with the right mix of organic substances. It is best to not source dirt from outside when it comes to indoor plants. Some herbs might differ in their soil requirements, but dirt is dirt, and you can worry about enhancing those aspects if your plants seem to need it.

In an outdoor garden, it is best to look at what you already have and find a way to enhance it instead of trying to replace a whole garden of soil. It can get very pricey. This might include adding manure to add nitrogen, or compost for other nutrients like calcium. If you have sandy soil, adding plant matter like wood chips can help the soil retain moisture, or adding lime can help neutralize overly acidic soil. Take a look at your food waste. This will most likely be a big enhancer in your garden. For example, tomatoes love crushed eggshells.

When you pot your plants, make sure that you put enough soil in the pot, that it is packed down enough that it can give the plant support, and that you bury the plant deep enough.

Water

All plants are a little different in their watering requirements. Over-watering can be just as bad, if not worse than, under-watering. Over-watering is often interpreted as using **too much** water, but it is actually watering *too frequently*. Some plants want their soil a little moist at all times, and some demand the soil dries between each watering. A great way to water potted plants is actually to fill a big pot of water and set your plant inside of it. It's better not to submerge the lip of the pot, so the dirt and plant don't lift. The drainage holes in the bottom of the pot will let in water from the bottom, and the plant will take as much as it wants. You will notice the level of water drop differently for each plant, as it takes what it needs. This prevents water on the plant, which reduces the chance of sunburn.

When watering, there is one more thing to remember. If you use town water, or if you live on a well with a water softener, your water might not be suitable for plants as is. Town water can be left in a watering can for about twenty-four hours before using—this will burn off any additives. You can also boil the water and let it cool, but this might burn off minerals in the water as well. Softened well water is done with salt, so if you have a faucet that is placed before the water softener process, it's best to fill your watering can with this instead. Distilled water is not beneficial to plants because it has no nutrients in it.

Sunlight

Plants need light to feed themselves, and it can be really difficult, inside and out, to have the right balance of sunlight. In the summer, plants that might typically be fairly tolerant to the sun can wither under a heatwave. Plants that need ten hours of direct sunlight a day might be just as dramatic if they only get nine and a half. Inside, you might find that some plants just won't cooperate on the windowsill. This issue can get worse in the winter, with less sunlight and a cold draft. Having a grow light, or even just converting an old lamp to supplement, can help push fussy plants through the winter, as well as boost the others. If you notice sunburn on your plant, it means it doesn't want as much direct sunlight. Moving it to a window that gets less light, typically a north-facing wall, can help.

Plant Tips

- If transplanting, make sure the plant is buried 1–3 inches below the soil level.
- Putting herbs in your kitchen can be a good way to remember to use them during the rush of cooking. Be careful to have them far enough away from heat, including steam.
- If you have tall plants, make sure you provide support through stakes, as well as making sure that the base of the stem is covered in enough dirt to make sure it has balance.
- Provide care and maintenance. This can be done by snipping and using the plant regularly to encourage growth.

Germinating: Starting Plants from Seed

If you are starting a garden, in or outside, you might choose to start it from seed. Seeds can be cheaper in-store, or you might have collected seeds from foraging. Starting from seed means that you are going to have to start your garden a bit earlier in the year, especially if you are transplanting to a garden outside. Being fairly north means that there is less of a growing season, especially if the plants are not native to the area. Starting them earlier means that you will match their peak growing time with peak season. Starting too late will mean they might not reach maturity before the end of the season. If the plant isn't slightly matured by the time it goes outside, it might not be strong enough to withstand colder mornings.

Common Mistakes

If you don't have a green thumb, that's okay. Plants seem simple, but the following are common mistakes to fix:

- Check the pot
- Check the location (sun, shade, cool drafts)
- Check the soil
- Over- and under-watering
- Planting seeds too deep or not deep enough
- Labeling seeds wrong
- Foragers and herbalists alike might be more hesitant to weed their gardens, as they know some common weeds are useful. If you choose to do this, make sure they don't take over your garden and pull the ones that you can't use to keep room for the ones you planted.

It might take some time to get the hang of home gardening. As you learn and grow, you will learn how to take care of plants without too much stress. The faster pace of learning, commitment, and responsibility of gardening in comparison to foraging, buying, and learning about herbs in general, can feel like a lot at once. You don't need to start a garden in your first year of practice, or at all if it doesn't suit you. But gardening will give you another perspective on plants. The work involved can impact how you see the food at the grocery store, or how you view the herbs you use in your remedies. The commitment to gardening can force us to learn quicker than we expected, even if we fail. Getting into the field at least once can force us to learn about what plants we need in our practice, what goes into a healthy plant, and even become more aware of our environment and ecosystem.

Those who struggle with gardening need to understand both sides of this argument. Gardening can seem really simple. It is, and it isn't. Gardening is not simple because it's not just dirt, sun, and water. The science behind growing plants is very complex, and without understanding that plants need a balance of all their environmental factors, you will not be able to provide care for these plants without looking at a manual each time. Gardening is simple once you understand how to balance these basics. Once the plant is in the soil, there is not much work besides making sure it's got water and it's happy.

Conclusion

Once you have entered the world of herbalism, you will always be a part of it. This knowledge is something that builds over time until you realize you are able to do a whole recipe without a reference or know exactly what herbs you need when you're feeling ill. The combination of self-learning in the field, along with safely sourced information, means that herbal healing can be safe and greatly beneficial when practiced the right way.

There are many plants that grow naturally throughout New England and the entire northeast. It can seem like an endless amount of knowledge to learn, but getting over the first curb of not knowing what you don't know is the hardest part. Starting with your local plants can really help you get a solid grip on herbalism without spending too much time or money. You don't need to know everything about every plant right away. Practicing through accurate harvesting and processing of fresh and dry herbs you slowly add to your inventory is the best way to ensure effective, long-term medical herbal practices.

There are an extensive number of ways to use these herbs internally, from simple teas to complex infusions. Externally, they can be simple compresses to multi-step salves. The methods of preparation of these herbs are just as varied as the recipes for making plant-based remedies to maintain holistic health. When in doubt, you can always buy herbs, but foraging can be more fun and fulfilling as you and your practice grow. For whatever reason, you might venture into gardening for more control over your supply.

A knowledgeable herbalist is one who is in charge of their own well-being through natural and holistic means. Start on your journey towards lifelong natural health, or continue your practice through better-honed specific skills.

References

Barotz, S., & Bilodeau, C. (2004). *Medicinal Plants of the Northeast.* bio.brandeis.edu.http://www.bio.brandeis.edu/fieldbio/medicinal_plants/pages/search_common.html

Bergeron, K. (n.d.). *Wild Herbs List of 70+ Medicinal Plant profiles.* Alternative Nature Online Herbal. https://altnature.com/gallery/index.html

*Complete List of Herbal Remedies for Common Ailments*Botanical Shaman. (n.d.). Retrieved January 25, 2022, from https://botanicalshaman.com/complete-list-of-herbal-remedies-for-common-ailments/

Editorial. (2020, July 2). *Medicinal plants index.* Botanical Online. https://www.botanical-online.com/en/medicinal-plants/medicinal-plants-index

Farmer's Almanac. (2022). *How to Start a Vegetable Garden.* https://www.almanac.com/sites/default/files/webform/pdf/almanac-start-a-garden.pdf

Freytag, C. (2019, February 5). 101 *Natural Remedies For Common Ailments.* Get Healthy U.

https://gethealthyu.com/101-natural-remedies-for-common-ailments/

Duke, Jame A. (2002). *Handbook of Medicinal Herbs*. https://www.enpab.it/images/2018/James_A._Duke_-_Handbook_of_Medicinal_Herbs.pdf

Herbal Recipes. (n.d.). Herbs with Rosalie. Retrieved January 25, 2022, from https://www.herbalremediesadvice.org/herbal-recipes.html

Mclean, R. (2020). *Foraging for Wild Plants*. https://www.nature.scot/sites/default/files/2020-03/Publication%202020%20-%20Foraging%20for%20Wild%20Plants.pdf

Medicinal Herbal Oil Recipes◻ - All information about healthy recipes and cooking tips. (n.d.). Www.therecipes.info. Retrieved January 25, 2022, from https://www.therecipes.info/medicinal-herbal-oil-recipes

Medicinal Herbs sorted by Herbs names. (n.d.). Herbs Natural. http://www.naturalmedicinalherbs.net/herbs/medicinal/

Medicinal Plants Pdf Recipes with ingredients, nutritions, instructions and related recipes. (n.d.). TfRecipes. Retrieved January 29, 2022, from https://www.tfrecipes.com/medicinal-plants-pdf/

Buhner, S. (2021, March 17). *Homemade Herbal Medicines for Common Ailments*. Mother Earth News. https://www.motherearthnews.com/natural-health/herbal-remedies/homemade-herbal-medicines-zm0z14fmzsor/

Nealley, E. (2020). *Medicinal Plants List.* Alderleaf Wilderness College. https://www.wildernesscollege.com/medicinal-plants-list.html

Poe, M. R., LeCompte, J., McLain, R., & Hurley, P. (2014). Urban foraging and the relational ecologies of belonging. *Social & Cultural Geography, 15*(8), 901–919. Taylor & Francis Online.

Starver, Mathew, et al. (2008). *Mistaken Identity? Invasive Plants and their Native Look-Alikes—an Identification Guide for the Mid-Atlantic.* www.nybg.org/files/scientists/rnaczi/Mistaken_Identity_Final.pdf

Plants Database. United States Department of Agriculture. Retrieved January 29, 2022, from

Weir, Kirsten. (2020, April 1) *Nurtured by .ature.* www.apa.org/monitor/2020/04/nurtured-nature.

Illustrations by Alina Levandovska

I hope you got value out of it.

I'm very open to feedback and always looking to improve.

Could you maybe share your opinion of the book in a few words?

I'd love to know what you think and see if there are areas you are interested in that I have not covered.

Made in the USA
Middletown, DE
01 July 2022